NCLEX-RN®
DRUG GUIDE

300 Medications You Need
to Know for the Exam
SIXTH EDITION

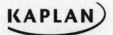

PUBLISHING

New York

Contributing Writer: Barbara H. Arnoldussen, RN, BS, MBA

© 2015, 2013, 2011, 2008, 2006, 2004 by Kaplan, Inc.

Published by Kaplan Publishing, a division of Kaplan, Inc.
750 Third Avenue
New York, NY 10017

10 9 8 7 6 5 4 3

ISBN 13: 978-1-62523-114-7

TABLE OF CONTENTS

TEN STEPS FOR MASTERING THE DRUGS ON THE NCLEX-RN EXAM

The best way to use this book to study for your nursing boards is to have a specific plan of attack! Then you can approach the sizeable task of learning about medications with confidence.

1. Get your mind set for future success.

Focus on the fact that, after you pass the NCLEX and become a licensed registered nurse (*not* "if you pass"), you will be using the information you learned in this book in your daily life, both personal and work.

You will be using drug information every day. Likewise, you need to study these go-to meds every day, even if it's only in short bursts. Don't rely on your previous experience of passing exams by pulling exhausting all-nighters. Do picture your study as gaining a solid understanding of concepts useful for your entire career.

2. Understand the book's flashcard format.

Think of the arrangement of information in this book as your two-sided master slide templates.

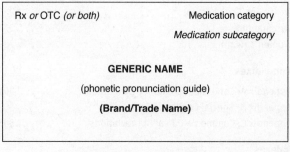

Front flashcard information

On the right-hand page, medications are arranged alphabetically under 22 drug categories. Each category tells which body system or medical condition the drug targets. Subcategories group drugs with similar desired action within that body system or for that medical condition.

For example, the first drug category, "Allergy and Asthma Medications," divides 10 medications under the following headings:

- Antihistamines (4 meds listed alphabetically by generic name)
- Corticosteroids (6 meds listed alphabetically by generic name)

To build a firm mental connection between medication facts, talk to yourself! First, pronounce the generic name while looking at the phonetic pronunciation guide. Then, say the generic name again, while looking at the medication category and subcategory. Engaging 3 learning channels at once (looking, talking, and listening) promotes active learning and enhances your recall.

Ignore the brand/trade name and the Rx or OTC notation. You won't need that information for the NCLEX!

Side Effects
First side effect
Second side effect, etc.

Nursing Considerations
- The purpose of giving the medication for a specific set of diseases or clinical conditions
- Other information about drug pharmacodynamics (how the human body responds to a drug) and pharmacokinetics (how a drug behaves in the human body)
- Key patient education highlights

Back flashcard information

On the upper lines of the left-hand page, the most common side effects are listed in roughly the order of occurrence. If self-care measures can prevent them, that patient-teaching opportunity is listed within the Nursing Considerations section.

The nursing profession is about action. Therefore, the most critical nursing implications for you to learn can be summarized as "go" or "no go" decisions for 2 situations:

- A vital sign such as pulse or respirations directs the nurse to withhold a medication (such as: no digoxin if the patient's pulse is under 60 beats per minute).
- A specific side effect signals a medical condition that is severe enough to warrant calling the health care provider immediately.

3. Keep your focus on the medication triangle.

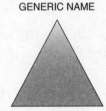

GENERIC NAME

PURPOSE   MEDICATION CATEGORY

Knowing the *purpose* for which the medication is designed allows you to accurately match patient and drug. It firmly links the drug to the mental connections you established on the front side, connecting the *generic name* with the *medication category*.

4. Calendar in chunks of time for formal study.

Plan on spending time with this book—but it doesn't have to happen all at once! This book is designed to be studied piecemeal. For example, if you want to review the whole book over 3 weeks, plan on a chapter a day. That lets you read the 22 chapters one drug category at a time.

5. Consider both paper and people companionship.

This small book has purposely been sized to fit into a purse or pocket. Take it with you everywhere you go—think of it as your new, rectangular BFF.

Waiting in line can become an opportunity to review one drug category. Counting down the minutes until the microwave rings is enough time to look at another drug category.

If you know a fellow student who is as motivated as you are, talk to them about setting up a "buddy system" where you can review your latest learning for each other. Make it a game: Quiz each other, *Jeopardy!* style, with one person giving the generic name and the other person guessing the purpose of that medication. You may be surprised by how these games energize you to prepare and remember.

6. Record your progress and thoughts.

By keeping track of your steps forward, you will enjoy 2 benefits: remembering where you left off, and marking the milestones of your journey. When you feel confident that you can recall the information up to a certain point in the book, mark it in some way that signals to you, "Done."

Make your messages to yourself obvious. What will communicate "Read here" or "Completed!" to you—a handwritten note? Folding over the corner of each completed page? Check marks in the margins? Remember: This is your book. Personalize it to work best for *you*.

Other additions that may help you focus on the material: circling or underlining key words, using a highlighter to enliven the facts you need with bright color, or mapping out similarities and differences of comparable medications in hand-drawn diagrams or tables. The more you interact with the material, the better you will be able to apply it.

7. Be alert for drug groupings.

The same suffix used in 2 or more medications hints at similarities in drug category and subcategory. Take the hint! As you go through the book, be alert for these "family" groupings, and chart them in your active study. Here is an example you can follow:

Suffix	Drug Category	Drug Subcategory	Generic Names
–afil	Genitourinary	Erectile dysfunction	Silden**afil** Tadal**afil** Varden**afil**
–asone	Allergy and asthma	Corticosteroids	Beclometh**asone** Flutic**asone** Momet**asone**
–azosin	Cardiovascular	Alpha blockers	Dox**azosin** Pr**azosin** Ter**azosin**
–cillin	Anti-infectives	Penicillins	Amoxi**cillin** Ampi**cillin** Peni**cillin**
–dipine	Cardiovascular	Calcium channel blockers	Amlo**dipine** Felo**dipine** Nife**dipine**
–olol	Cardiovascular	Beta blockers	Aten**olol** Metopr**olol** Propran**olol**
–pam	Mental health	Antianxiety	Diaze**pam** Loraze**pam** Citalop**ram**

Suffix	Drug Category	Drug Subcategory	Generic Names
–pril	Cardiovascular	ACE inhibitors	Benaze**pril** Capto**pril** Enala**pril** Lisino**pril** Rami**pril**
–romycin	Anti-infectives	Macrolides	Azith**romycin** Clarith**romycin** Eryth**romycin**
–statin	Cardiovascular	Antilipemic	Atorva**statin** Fluva**statin** Lova**statin** Prava**statin** Rosuva**statin** Simva**statin**
–tidine	Gastrointestinal	Antiulcer	Cime**tidine** Famo**tidine** Rani**tidine**
–vir	Anti-infectives	Antiviral	Acyclo**vir** Oseltami**vir** Valacyclo**vir**

8. Don't worry about brand names.

You are unlikely to see any trade/brand names on your NCLEX. The National Council on State Boards of Nursing, which develops the exam, strives for consistency over time—a stance that favors either the generic name or the drug category/subcategory. Trade and brand names are at the discretion of the many pharmaceutical manufacturing companies that produce them. *Trade and brand names can change.* Generic names are more stable, and thus are favored by the National Council.

9. Take a quick final review.

Shortly before test day, pick up this book once again. Even if you only have the opportunity to look at the table of contents, doing so will refresh your memory before you take the NCLEX.

10. Get ready to celebrate!

Once you've passed the exam, keep this book as a souvenir of that fact that you earned your place in the ranks of registered nurses!

CETIRIZINE HCL
(se-<u>teer</u>-a-zeen)

(Zyrtec)

• •

FEXOFENADINE
(fex-oh-<u>fen</u>-a-deen)

(Allegra)

Side Effects

Drowsiness	Diarrhea	Stomach pain
Dry mouth	Fatigue	Vomiting

Nursing Considerations

- Relief of seasonal allergic rhinitis symptoms
- Relief of perennial allergic rhinitis caused by molds, animal dander, and other allergens
- Avoid alcohol during cetirizine therapy
- Call physician immediately for difficulty breathing or swallowing
- Notify physician for hydroxyzine (Vistaril) allergy
- Rx

• •

Side Effects

Drowsiness	Pain	Difficulty breathing
Headache	Cough	Hoarseness
Dizziness	Hives	Swelling
Diarrhea	Rash	
Vomiting	Itching	

Nursing Considerations

- Management of rhinitis, allergy symptoms, chronic idiopathic urticaria
- Avoid alcohol, CNS depressants
- 60 mg tablet: onset within 1 hour, peak 2–3 hours, duration about 12 hours
- 180 mg tablet: duration 24 hours
- Notify physician if taking erythromycin or ketoconazole (Nizoral)
- If taking aluminum magnesium antacid, take antacid a few hours before or after fexofenadine
- Rx

HYDROXYZINE
(hye-<u>drox</u>-i-zeen)

(Atarax, Vistaril)

• •

LORATADINE
(lor-<u>a</u>-ti-deen)

(Alavert, Claritin)

SIDE EFFECTS

Drowsiness	Dizziness	Chest congestion
Dry mouth, nose, and throat	Headache	Reddening of skin

NURSING CONSIDERATIONS

- Treatment of pruritus, pre-op anxiety, post-op nausea and vomiting, to potentiate opioid analgesics, sedation
- PO: onset 15–30 minutes, duration 4–6 hours
- Avoid use with alcohol, CNS depressants
- Teach patient that dizziness/drowsiness may occur; use caution in potentially hazardous activities
- Treatment of symptoms of alcohol withdrawal
- Notify physician of diagnosis of glaucoma, ulcers, enlarged prostate gland, liver disease, hypertension, seizures, or hyperthyroidism
- Observe for difficulty breathing
- Muscle weakness
- Increased anxiety
- Rx

• •

SIDE EFFECTS

Headache	Nervousness	Swelling of face or extremities
Dry mouth	Weakness	Hoarseness
Epistaxis (nosebleed)	Stomach pain	Mouth sores
Sore throat	Wheezing	Insomnia
Diarrhea	Dysphagia	
Rash	Dyspnea	
	Hives	

NURSING CONSIDERATIONS

- Management of seasonal rhinitis
- Avoid alcohol, CNS depressants
- Take on empty stomach 1 hour before or 2 hours after meals
- Onset 1–3 hours, peak 8–12 hours, duration ≥24 hours
- OTC, Rx

BECLOMETHASONE
(be-kloe-<u>meth</u>-a-sone)

(Beclovent, Beconase)

• •

FLUNISOLIDE
(floo-<u>niss</u>-oh-lide)

(Aerobid, Nasalide)

SIDE EFFECTS

Dysphonia
Hoarseness
Oropharyngeal fungal infections
Headache
Sore throat
Dyspepsia

Unpleasant taste and smell
Rhinitis
Nausea
Cough
Angioedema
Back pain

NURSING CONSIDERATIONS

- Used in chronic asthma treatment, seasonal or perennial rhinitis
- Prevention of recurrence of nasal polyps after surgical removal
- Nasal spray: onset 5–7 days (up to 3 weeks in some patients), peak up to 3 weeks
- Inhaler: onset 10 minutes
- Use regular peak flow monitoring to determine respiratory status
- Rx

• •

SIDE EFFECTS

Dysphonia
Hoarseness
Oropharyngeal
  fungal infections
Headache

Sore throat
Nasal congestion,
  cold symptoms
Nausea, vomiting,
  diarrhea

Unpleasant taste,
  upset stomach
Epistaxis
  (nosebleed)

NURSING CONSIDERATIONS

- Used in chronic asthma treatment, seasonal or perennial rhinitis
- Onset: few days
- Use regular peak flow monitoring to determine respiratory status
- Rx

FLUTICASONE
(floo-<u>tik</u>-a-sone)

(Flonase)

• •

FLUTICASONE PROPIONATE SALMETEROL
(floo-<u>tik</u>-a-sone <u>proe</u>-pee-oh-nate sal-<u>meh</u>-te-role)

(Advair Diskus)

SIDE EFFECTS

Dysphonia

Hoarseness

Oropharyngeal fungal infections

Headache

Sore throat

Nasal congestion, cold symptoms

Nausea, vomiting, diarrhea

Unpleasant taste, upset stomach

Epistaxis (nosebleed), nasal irritation

Hives

Dyspnea

Dysphagia

Angioedema

NURSING CONSIDERATIONS

- Used in chronic asthma treatment, seasonal or perennial rhinitis
- Nasal spray: onset within 2 days, peak 1–2 weeks
- Use regular peak flow monitoring to determine respiratory status
- Rx

• •

SIDE EFFECTS

Nausea, vomiting, diarrhea

Headache

Dysphonia, hoarseness

Throat irritation, cough

Oropharyngeal fungal infections

Muscle and bone pain

Viral respiratory infections, bronchitis

NURSING CONSIDERATIONS

- Used when asthma is not well controlled with long-term inhaled corticosteroids; COPD
- Oral inhalation; rinse mouth with water after inhalation
- Twice-daily dosage, 12 hours apart; used long term
- Use regular peak flow monitoring to determine respiratory status
- Monitor growth of pediatric patient
- Monitor for glaucoma and cataracts
- May decrease bone mineral density
- Monitor for eosinophilic conditions, hypokalemia, and hyperglycemia
- May increase risk of pneumonia in patients with COPD
- May cause worsening of infections
- Check oral cavity for Candida albicans
- Rx

MOMETASONE

(moe-<u>met</u>-a-sone)

(Nasonex Spray)

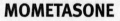

TRIAMCINOLONE

(try-am-<u>sin</u>-oh-lone)

(Nasacort AQ Spray)

SIDE EFFECTS

Dysphonia
Hoarseness
Oropharyngeal fungal infections
Headache
Sore throat

Nasal congestion, cold
  symptoms
Nausea, vomiting, diarrhea
Unpleasant taste, upset stomach

NURSING CONSIDERATIONS

- Used in chronic asthma treatment, seasonal or perennial rhinitis
- Nasal spray: onset few days, peak up to 3 weeks
- Use regular peak flow monitoring to determine respiratory status
- Rx

• •

SIDE EFFECTS

Dysphonia; hoarseness
Oropharyngeal fungal infections
Headache
Sore throat
Nasal congestion, cold
  symptoms

Nausea, vomiting, diarrhea
Unpleasant taste, upset stomach
Epistaxis (nosebleed)
Flu syndrome
Increased cough
Bronchitis

NURSING CONSIDERATIONS

- Used in chronic asthma treatment, seasonal or perennial rhinitis
- Nasal spray: onset few days, peak 3–4 days
- PO/IM: peak 1–2 hours
- Use regular peak flow monitoring to determine respiratory status
- Rx

ACETAMINOPHEN
(a-seet-a-<u>min</u>-a-fen)

(Tylenol)

• •

ACETAMINOPHEN/ASPIRIN/CAFFEINE
(a-seet-a-<u>min</u>-a-fen/<u>as</u>-pir-in/kaf-<u>een</u>)

(Excedrin)

SIDE EFFECTS

Anemia (long-term use)   Angioedema
Liver and kidney failure   Hives, itching
Dyspnea (prolonged high doses)

NURSING CONSIDERATIONS

- Treatment of mild pain or fever
- PO: onset less than 1 hour, peak 30 minutes to 2 hours, duration 4–6 hours
- Rectal: onset slow, peak 1–2 hours, duration 3–4 hours
- Take crushed or whole with full glass of water
- Can give with food or milk to decrease GI upset
- Signs of chronic poisoning: rapid, weak pulse; dyspnea; cold, clammy extremities
- Signs of chronic overdose: bleeding, bruising, malaise, fever, sore throat, anorexia, jaundice
- OTC

• •

SIDE EFFECTS

Upset stomach,   Depressed mood,   Insomnia
  heartburn   anxious or restless
                        feelings

NURSING CONSIDERATIONS

- Management of mild to moderate pain or fever
- Do not give to children or teenagers with fever, flu symptoms, or chickenpox; Reye syndrome may develop
- Watch out for symptoms of stomach bleeding or liver problems

ASPIRIN
(<u>as</u>-pir-in)

· ·

CELECOXIB
(sel-eh-<u>cox</u>-ib)

(Celebrex)

SIDE EFFECTS

Nausea, vomiting	Dyspnea	GI bleeding
Rash	Melena	
Angioedema	Tinnitus	

NURSING CONSIDERATIONS

- Management of mild to moderate pain or fever, transient ischemic attacks, prophylaxis of MI, ischemic stroke, angina
- PO: onset 15–30 minutes, peak 1–2 hours, duration 4–6 hours
- Rectal: onset slow, 20%–60% absorbed if retained 2–4 hours
- With long-term use, check for liver damage: dark urine, clay-colored stools, yellowing of skin and sclera, itching, abdominal pain, fever, diarrhea
- For arthritis, give 30 minutes before exercise; may take 2 weeks before full effect is felt
- Discard tablets if vinegar-like smell
- Do not give to children or teens with flulike symptoms or chickenpox; Reye syndrome may develop
- OTC

• •

SIDE EFFECTS

Fatigue	dry mouth,	Back pain
Anxiety, depression, nervousness	constipation	Tachycardia
	Angioedema	Jaundice
Nausea, vomiting, anorexia,	Hives	Dysuria
	Dyspnea	

NURSING CONSIDERATIONS

- Management of acute, chronic arthritis pain and primary dysmenorrheal pain relief within 60 minutes
- Onset: 24–48 hours, duration 12–24 hours
- Can take without regard to meals
- Increasing doses do not appear to increase effectiveness
- Do not take if allergic to sulfonamides, aspirin, or NSAIDs
- Rx

IBUPROFEN
(eye-byoo-<u>proe</u>-fen)

(Advil, Motrin IB)

• •

NAPROXEN
(na-<u>prox</u>-en)

(Aleve [OTC], Naprosyn)

SIDE EFFECTS

Headache
Tinnitus
Nausea, anorexia
Dizziness

Blood dyscrasias
Constipation
GI bleeding

NURSING CONSIDERATIONS

- Treatment of rheumatoid arthritis, osteoarthritis, primary dysmenorrhea, gout, dental pain, musculoskeletal disorders, fever
- Onset: 30 minutes, peak 1–2 hours
- Contact clinician if ringing or roaring in ears, which may indicate toxicity
- Contact clinician if changes in urinary pattern, increased weight, edema, increased pain in joints, fever, or blood in urine, which may indicate kidney damage
- Use sunscreen to prevent photosensitivity
- Avoid use with ASA, NSAIDs, and alcohol, which may precipitate
- GI bleeding
- Avoid use with anticoagulants
- May have an increased risk of MI or stroke
- OTC, Rx

• •

SIDE EFFECTS

GI bleeding
Blood dyscrasias
Tinnitus
Headache

Insomnia
Vision changes
Rash
Angioedema

Jaundice
Tachycardia
Back pain
Nausea

NURSING CONSIDERATIONS

- Management of mild to moderate pain
- Treatment of rheumatoid, juvenile, and gouty arthritis; osteoarthritis; primary dysmenorrhea
- Patients with asthma, ASA hypersensitivity, or nasal polyps have increased risk of hypersensitivity
- Contact clinician if blurred vision or ringing or roaring in ears, which may indicate toxicity
- Contact clinician if black stools, flulike symptoms
- Contact clinician if changes in urinary pattern, increased weight, edema, increased pain in joints, fever, or blood in urine, which may indicate kidney damage
- Avoid use with ASA, steroids, and alcohol
- May increase risk of MI or stroke
- OTC, Rx

CODEINE
(<u>koe</u>-deen)

· ·

HYDROCODONE BITARTRATE/ ACETAMINOPHEN
(hye-droe-<u>koe</u>-doan)

(Lortab, Vicodin)

SIDE EFFECTS

Drowsiness, sedation

Nausea, vomiting, anorexia

Respiratory depression

Constipation

Orthostatic hypotension

Dysuria

Hives

Dyspnea

Syncope

Angioedema

Seizures

NURSING CONSIDERATIONS

- Treatment of moderate to severe pain, nonproductive cough
- PO: onset 30–45 minutes, peak 60–120 minutes, duration 4–6 hours
- IM/subQ: onset 10–30 minutes, peak 30–60 minutes, duration 4–6 hours
- Do not give if respirations are less than 12 per minute
- Avoid use with alcohol, CNS depressants
- Withdrawal symptoms may occur: nausea, vomiting, cramps, fever, faintness, anorexia
- Physical dependency may result from long-term use
- Rx C-II, III, IV, V (depends on route)

• •

SIDE EFFECTS

Dizziness

Drowsiness

Constipation

Nausea

Vomiting

Respiratory depression

Sedation

Impairment of mental and physical performance

Rash

Pruritus

NURSING CONSIDERATIONS

- Used for relief of moderate to moderately severe pain
- Use with CNS depressants and/or alcohol may result in addictive CNS depression
- May be habit-forming
- Avoid alcohol during treatment
- Use with caution in patients with pulmonary considerations
- Rx C-III

HYDROMORPHONE
(hye-droe-<u>mor</u>-fone)

(Dilaudid)

• •

MEPERIDINE
(me-<u>pair</u>-i-deen)

(Demerol)

SIDE EFFECTS

Drowsiness, sedation
Nausea, vomiting, anorexia
Respiratory depression
Constipation, cramps

Orthostatic hypotension
Confusion, headache
Rash

NURSING CONSIDERATIONS

- Treatment of moderate to severe pain, nonproductive cough
- PO: onset 15–30 minutes, peak 30–60 minutes, duration 4–6 hours
- IM: onset 15 minutes, peak 30–60 minutes, duration 4–5 hours
- IV: onset 10–15 minutes, peak 15–30 minutes, duration 2–3 hours
- subQ: onset 15 minutes, peak 30–90 minutes, duration 4 hours
- Rectal: duration 6–8 hours
- Do not give if respirations are less than 12 per minute
- Avoid use with alcohol, CNS depressants
- Withdrawal symptoms may occur: nausea, vomiting, cramps, fever, faintness, anorexia
- Physical dependency may result from long-term use
- Elderly patients may require lower doses
- Rx C-II

• •

SIDE EFFECTS

Drowsiness,
sedation
Respiratory
depression
Euphoria

Orthostatic
hypotension
Confusion,
headache
Bradycardia

Diaphoresis
Urticaria

NURSING CONSIDERATIONS

- Management of moderate to severe pain, pre-op sedation, post-op, and OB analgesia
- PO: onset 10–15 minutes, peak 30–60 minutes, duration 2–4 hours (usually 3)
- IM: onset 10–15 minutes, peak 30–50 minutes, duration 2–4 hours (usually 3)
- IV: onset less than 5 minutes, peak 5-7 minutes, duration 2–4 hours (usually 3)
- subQ: onset 10–15 minutes, peak 30–50 minutes, duration 2–4 hours (usually 3)
- Do not give if respirations are less than 12 per minute
- Avoid use with alcohol, CNS depressants
- Withdrawal symptoms may occur: nausea, vomiting, cramps, fever, faintness, anorexia
- Physical dependency may result from long-term use
- Do not co-infuse with barbiturates, aminophylline, heparin, morphine, methicillin, phenytoin, sodium bicarbonate, sulfadiazine, or sulfisoxazole
- Rx C-II

METHADONE
(<u>meth</u>-a-doan)

(Dolophine, Methadose)

• •

MORPHINE
(<u>mor</u>-feen)

(MS Contin)

SIDE EFFECTS

Drowsiness,
sedation
Nausea, vomiting,
anorexia
Respiratory
depression

Constipation,
cramps
Orthostatic
hypotension
Confusion,
headache
Rash

Arrhythmias
Syncope
Agitation
Diaphoresis
Hypokalemia
Pulmonary edema

NURSING CONSIDERATIONS

- Relief of pain, detoxification/maintenance of narcotic addiction
- PO: onset 30–60 minutes, peak 30–60 minutes, duration 4–6 hours (with continuous dosing, duration of action may increase to 22 to 48 hours)
- Do not give if respirations are less than 12 per minute
- Avoid use with alcohol, CNS depressants
- Withdrawal symptoms may occur: nausea, vomiting, cramps, fever, faintness, anorexia
- Physical dependency may result from long-term use
- Rx C-II

• •

SIDE EFFECTS

Respiratory
depression
Sedation

Euphoria
Orthostatic
hypotension

Bradycardia
Diaphoresis
Urticaria

NURSING CONSIDERATIONS

- Management of severe pain
- Continuous dosing is more effective than prn; may be given by patientcontrolled analgesia (PCA)
- PO: onset 15–60 minutes, peak 30–60 minutes, duration 3–6 hours
- IM: onset 10–15 minutes, peak 30–50 minutes, duration 2–4 hours (usually 3)
- IV: onset less than 5 minutes, peak 18 minutes, duration 3–6 hours
  subQ: onset 10–15 minutes, peak 30–50 minutes, duration 2–4 hours (usually 3)
- Withdrawal symptoms may occur: nausea, vomiting, cramps, fever, faintness, anorexia
- Physical dependency may result from long-term use
- Monitor for increased respiratory and CNS depression when given with cimetidine, clomipramine, nortriptyline, or amitriptyline
- Rx C-II

OXYCODONE
(ox-i-<u>koe</u>-doan)

(OxyContin; with aspirin Percodan, with acetaminophen Percocet)

• •

DABIGATRAN ETEXILATE
(da-bi-<u>ga</u>-tran e-<u>tex</u>-i-late)

(Pradaxa)

SIDE EFFECTS

Drowsiness, sedation

Nausea, vomiting, anorexia

Respiratory depression

Constipation, cramps

Confusion, headache

Rash

Euphoria

Urinary retention

Orthostatic hypotension

NURSING CONSIDERATIONS

- Management of moderate to severe pain
- PO: peak 30–60 minutes, duration 4–6 hours
- Controlled-release: peak 3–4 minutes, duration 12 hours
- Do not give if respirations are less than 12 per minute
- Avoid use with alcohol, CNS depressants
- Withdrawal symptoms may occur: nausea, vomiting, cramps, fever, faintness, anorexia
- Physical dependency may result from long-term use
- Rx C-II

• •

SIDE EFFECTS

Dyspepsia

Abdominal discomfort

Epigastric pain

GI hemorrhage

Bleeding

Hematoma

Anemia

NURSING CONSIDERATIONS

- Used for prevention of stroke in patients with nonvalvular atrial fibrillation
- Keep in original packaging (blister pack or manufacturer bottle) until administered
- PO: may take without regard to meals
- Do not crush or chew capsules
- Closely monitor for signs of bleeding
- Increased risk of bleeding when combined with aspirin, other antiplatelets, or anticoagulants
- Reduced dose required in renally impaired patients
- Stop med 24 hours before surgery
- Rx

ENOXAPARIN

(ee-noks-a-<u>par</u>-in)

(Lovenox)

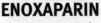

HEPARIN

(<u>hep</u>-a-rin)

SIDE EFFECTS

Bleeding

Bruising

Injection site hematoma

Injection site ecchymosis

Hematuria

Increase in AST/ALT

NURSING CONSIDERATIONS

- Anticoagulation during acute coronary syndromes, prophylaxis and treatment of venous thromboembolism
- Injection: subQ; can be given IV during cardiac procedures
- Do not use in patients with a history of heparin-induced thrombocytopenia
- Use with caution in patients with impaired renal function or morbid obesity
- Monitor closely for signs of bleeding or excessive bruising
- Stop med 12–24 hours before surgery
- Rx

• •

SIDE EFFECTS

Can produce hemorrhage from any body site (10%)

Tissue irritation/pain at injection site

Anemia

Thrombocytopenia

Fever

NURSING CONSIDERATIONS

- Prophylaxis and treatment of thromboembolic disorders in very low doses (10–100 units) to maintain patency of IV catheters (heparin flush)
- Therapeutic PTT @ 1.5–2.5 times the control without signs of hemorrhage
- IV: peak 5 minutes, duration 2–6 hours (give over 1 minute)
- Injection: give deep subQ; never IM (danger of hematoma), onset 20–60 minutes, duration 8–12 hours
- Antidote: protamine sulfate within 30 minutes
- Signs of hemorrhage: bleeding gums, epistaxis (nosebleed), unusual bleeding, black or tarry stools, hematuria, fall in hematocrit or blood pressure, guaiac-positive stools
- Avoid ASA-containing products and NSAIDs
- Wear medical information tag
- Abrupt withdrawal may precipitate increased coagulability
- Rx

RIVAROXABAN

(riv-a-<u>rox</u>-a-ban)

(Xarelto)

• •

WARFARIN

(<u>war</u>-far-in)

(Coumadin)

SIDE EFFECTS

Bleeding	Peripheral edema	Hematoma
Bruising	Nausea	Anemia
Epistaxis	Dyspepsia	Thrombocytopenia

NURSING CONSIDERATIONS

- Stroke prevention in nonvalvular atrial fibrillation, prevention and treatment of venous thromboembolism
- Dose reduction required in renal impairment
- PO: give doses >15 mg with food; lower doses may be given without regard to food
- Stop med 24 hours before surgery
- Monitor closely for signs of bleeding or excessive bruising
- Rx

• •

SIDE EFFECTS

Hemorrhage	Syncope	Elevated liver enzymes
Diarrhea	Anemia	
Rash	Dermatitis	Anaphylactic reactions
Fever	Jaundice	
Angina syndrome		

NURSING CONSIDERATIONS

- Management of pulmonary emboli, deep vein thrombosis, MI, atrial dysrhythmias, postcardiac valve replacement
- Therapeutic PT @ 1.5–2.5 times the control, INR @ 2.0–3.0
- Onset: 12–24 hours, peak 1.5 to 3 days; duration 3 to 5 days
- Avoid foods high in vitamin K: many green leafy vegetables
- Do not interchange brands; potencies may not be equivalent
- Do not take any drug or herb without physician approval—may change effect
- Avoid ASA-containing products and NSAIDs
- Oral anticoagulants may cause red-orange discoloration of alkaline urine, interfering with some lab tests
- Wear medical information tag
- Rx

CARBAMAZEPINE
(kar-ba-<u>maz</u>-e-peen)

(Carbatrol, Tegretol)

• •

DIVALPROEX SODIUM
(dye-<u>val</u>-proe-ex)

(Depakote, Depakote ER)

SIDE EFFECTS

Myelosuppression

Dizziness, drowsiness

Ataxia

Diplopia, rash

Photosensitivity

Depression

Nausea

Vomiting

Dyspepsia

Aplastic anemia

Stevens-Johnson syndrome

Suicide attempts in bipolar patients

NURSING CONSIDERATIONS

- Management of seizures, trigeminal neuralgia, diabetic neuropathy
- Avoid driving and other activities requiring alertness the first 3 days
- Monitor blood levels, CBC regularly, esp. during first 2 months; periodic eye exams
- Take with food or milk to decrease GI upset; tablets (nonextendedrelease) may be crushed, extended-release capsules may be opened and mixed with juice or soft food (no grapefruit products)
- Urine may turn pink to brown
- Avoid abrupt withdrawal; discontinue gradually
- Avoid use with alcohol, CNS depressants
- Inform physician before taking any new medication or herbal medication
- Rx

• •

SIDE EFFECTS

Sedation, drowsiness, dizziness

Mental status and behavioral changes

Nausea, vomiting, constipation, diarrhea

Heartburn

Prolonged bleeding time

Hepatotoxicity

Teratogenicity

Pancreatitis

Thrombocytopenia

Headache

Diplopia

Tremor

Alopecia

Multiorgan hypersensitivity

NURSING CONSIDERATIONS

- Management of seizures, manic episodes assoc. with bipolar disorder (delayed-release only), migraine prophylaxis (delayed- and extendedrelease only)
- Take with or immediately after meals to lessen GI upset; swallow whole
- Avoid abrupt withdrawal after long-term use; discontinue gradually to prevent convulsions
- Monitor blood levels, platelets, bleeding time, and liver function tests
- Delayed-release products: peak blood level 3–5 hours, duration 12–24 hours
- Extended-release products: onset 2–4 days, peak blood level 7–14 hours, duration 24 hours
- Wear medical information tag
- Rx

GABAPENTIN
(ga-ba-pen-tin)

(Gabarone, Neurontin)

· ·

Anticonvulsants
Anticonvulsants

LAMOTRIGINE
(la-moe-tri-jeen)

(Lamictal)

SIDE EFFECTS

Drowsiness	Constipation	Back or joint pain
Ataxia	Memory problems	Edema
Diplopia	Uncontrolled	Flulike symptoms
Rhinitis	shaking	Seizures

NURSING CONSIDERATIONS

- Used for management of seizures and postherpetic neuralgia, diabetic neuropathy
- Do not take within 2 hours of antacid use
- Avoid abrupt withdrawal after long-term use; discontinue gradually over a week to prevent convulsions
- Give without regard to meals; can open capsules and put in juice or applesauce
- Do not crush or chew capsules
- Use caution with hazardous activities
- Wear medical information tag
- Rx

• •

SIDE EFFECTS

Ataxia, dizziness	Loss of coordination
Headache	Mood changes
Nausea, vomiting, anorexia	Irritability
Diplopia, blurred vision	Insomnia
Abdominal pain, dysmenorrhea	Depression

NURSING CONSIDERATIONS

- Used for management of seizures, abnormal mood disorders
- In pediatric patients, stop at first sign of rash; all patients should notify clinician of rashes
- Take divided doses with meals or just after to decrease adverse effects
- Use caution with hazardous activities until stabilized
- Avoid abrupt withdrawal; stop gradually to prevent increase in frequency of seizures
- Wear medical information tag
- Rx

PHENOBARBITAL

(fee-noe-<u>bar</u>-bi-tal)

(Luminal)

· ·

PHENYTOIN

(<u>fen</u>-i-toyn)

(Dilantin)

SIDE EFFECTS

Drowsiness, lethargy, rash
GI upset
Initially constricts pupils
Respiratory depression
Ataxia

Nightmares
Unusual bleeding
Dyspnea
Dysphagia
Excitement in children

NURSING CONSIDERATIONS

- Management of epilepsy, febrile seizures in children, sedation, insomnia
- IV: slow rate—resuscitation equipment should be available
- IM: inject deep into large muscle mass to prevent tissue sloughing, can give subQ, onset 10–30 minutes
- PO: onset 20–60 minutes, peak 8–12 hours, duration 6–10 hours
- Use caution with hazardous activities until stabilized; drowsiness usually diminishes after initial weeks of therapy
- Nystagmus may indicate early toxicity
- Long-term use withdrawal symptoms: vomiting, sweating, abdomen/muscle cramps, tremors, and possibly convulsions
- Vitamin D supplements are indicated for long-term use
- Rx C-IV

• •

SIDE EFFECTS

Drowsiness, ataxia
Nystagmus
Blurred vision
Hirsutism

Lethargy
GI upset
Gingival
   hypertrophy

Suicidal behavior
Skin rash

NURSING CONSIDERATIONS

- Management of seizures, migraines, trigeminal neuralgia, Bell's palsy
- PO: take divided doses, with or immediately after meals, to decrease adverse effects
- May color urine and sweat pink/red/brown
- May cause increase in blood sugar
- IV administration may lead to cardiac arrest—have resuscitation equipment available; never mix in IV with any other drug or dextrose
- Avoid abrupt withdrawal to prevent convulsions
- Do not use antacids or antidiarrheals within 2 hours of med
- Use caution with hazardous activities until stabilized
- Folic acid supplements are indicated for long-term use
- Wear medical information tag
- Rx

PREGABALIN
(pre-gab-a-lin)

(Lyrica)

• •

TOPIRAMATE
(toh-pyre-ah-mate)

(Topamax, Topiragen)

SIDE EFFECTS

Dizziness, tiredness, weakness

Headache

Nausea, vomiting, constipation

Flatulence, bloating

Mental status and behavioral changes

Anxiety

Lack of coordination, loss of balance, unsteadiness

Uncontrollable shaking or jerking of a part of the body, muscle twitching

Increased appetite, weight gain

Swelling of the arms, hands, feet, ankles, or lower legs

Back pain

Infection

Angioedema

Neuropathy

NURSING CONSIDERATIONS

- Treatment for neuropathic pain, diabetic pain, pain after shingles, partial onset seizures in adults with epilepsy who already take one or more drugs for seizures
- Take around the same time every day, 2–3 times daily; full therapeutic effects may require 4 weeks
- Avoid abrupt withdrawal after long-term use; discontinue gradually
- Avoid use with alcohol
- Use caution in potentially hazardous activities
- May increase the risk of suicidal thoughts or behavior
- Rx

• •

SIDE EFFECTS

Dizziness, drowsiness, fatigue

Impaired concentration/memory

Nervousness, speech problems

Nausea, weight loss

Vision problems

Ataxia

Photosensitivity

Behavior problems, mood problems

Anorexia

NURSING CONSIDERATIONS

- Used for management of seizures, prophylaxis of migraine headache, cluster headache, bulimia
- Give without regard to meals; can open capsules and put in juice or applesauce Avoid abrupt withdrawal after long-term use; discontinue gradually to prevent seizures and status epilepticus
- Use caution with hazardous activities until stabilized
- Increase fluid intake to prevent formation of kidney stones
- Stop drug immediately if eye problems; could lead to permanent loss of vision
- Use sunscreen and protective clothing to prevent photosensitivity
- Wear medical information tag
- Rx

VALPROATE
(val-<u>proe</u>-ate)

(Depacon)

• •

VALPROIC ACID
(val-<u>proe</u>-ic)

(Depakene, Myproic Acid)

SIDE EFFECTS

Sedation, drowsiness, dizziness

Mental status and behavioral changes

Nausea, vomiting, constipation, diarrhea, heartburn

Prolonged bleeding time

Hepatotoxicity

Teratogenicity

Pancreatitis

NURSING CONSIDERATIONS

- Used for management of seizures, manic episodes associated
- with bipolar disorders, prevent migraines
- Avoid abrupt withdrawal after long-term use; discontinue gradually to prevent convulsions
- May be given with food to decrease GI irritation
- Monitor blood levels, platelets, bleeding time, and liver function tests
- Onset of anticonvulsant effect: 2–4 days, peak blood level at end of infusion, duration 6–24 hours
- Rx

• •

SIDE EFFECTS

Sedation, drowsiness, dizziness

Mental status and behavioral changes

Nausea, vomiting, constipation, diarrhea, heartburn

Prolonged bleeding time

Hepatotoxicity

Teratogenicity

Pancreatitis

NURSING CONSIDERATIONS

- Used for management of seizures, mania, prevent migraine headaches
- Take with or immediately after meals to lessen GI upset
- Swallow capsules whole (no crushing, chewing)
- Avoid abrupt withdrawal after long-term use; discontinue gradually to prevent convulsions
- Monitor blood levels, platelets, bleeding time, and liver function tests
- Onset: 2–4 days, peak blood level of syrup 15–120 minutes, of capsules 1–4 hours, duration 6–24 hours (varies with age)
- Wear medical information tag
- Rx

AMIKACIN, GENTAMICIN, TOBRAMYCIN

(am-i-<u>kay</u>-sin, jen-ta-<u>mye</u>-sin,
toe-bra-<u>mye</u>-sin)

(Amikin, Garamycin, Tobrex)

. . . .

AMPHOTERICIN B

(am-foe-<u>tair</u>-i-sin)

(Abelcet, Amphotec, Fungizone)

SIDE EFFECTS

Use during pregnancy can result in bilateral congenital deafness

Ototoxicity cranial nerve VIII

Nephrotoxicity

Allergic reaction: fever, difficulty breathing, rash

Vertigo, tinnitus

NURSING CONSIDERATIONS

- Treatment of severe systemic infections of CNS, respiratory, GI, urinary tract, bone, skin, soft tissues, acute PID
- IV over 30 minutes to 1 hour; IM by deep, slow injection, never subQ
- Careful monitoring of blood levels
- Check peak—2 hours after med given
- Check trough—at time of dose/prior to med
- Monitor for signs of superinfection (diarrhea, URI, coated tongue)
- Immediately report hearing or balance problems
- Encourage fluids to 8–10 glasses/day
- Rx

• •

SIDE EFFECTS

Blood, kidney, heart, liver abnormalities

GI upset

Hypokalemiain-duced muscle pain

CNS disturbances, inefficient hearing

Skin irritation and thrombosis if IV infiltrates

Rash

Fever

Malaise

Hypotension

Headache

Nephrotoxicity

NURSING CONSIDERATIONS

- Treatment of histoplasmosis, skin infections, septicemia, meningitis in HIV patients
- Do not mix with other drugs
- Monitor vital signs; report fever or change in function, especially nervous system
- Check for hypokalemia
- Meticulous care and observation of injection site
- Potential benefits must be balanced against serious side effects
- Rx

FLUCONAZOLE
(flew-<u>kon</u>-uh-zol)

(Diflucan)

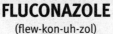

Anti-Infectives
Antimalarials

HYDROXYCHLOROQUINE
(hye-drox-ee-<u>klor</u>-oh-kween)

(Plaquenil)

SIDE EFFECTS

Nausea	Diarrhea
Headache	Taste distortion
Abdominal pain	

NURSING CONSIDERATIONS

- Used to treat vaginal, esophageal, or systemic candidiasis; cryptococcal meningitis
- Prothrombin time is increased after warfarin usage
- Take missed dose as soon as noticed, but do not double dose
- Reduces metabolism of tolbutamide, glyburide, and glipizide
- Glucose levels should be monitored, especially in diabetics
- Rx

. . . .

SIDE EFFECTS

Eye disturbances	Rash
Nausea, vomiting	Headache
Anorexia	Loss of hair

NURSING CONSIDERATIONS

- Management of malaria, lupus erythematosus, rheumatoid arthritis
- Peak 1–2 hours
- Take at the same time each day to maintain blood level
- Give with meats to decrease GI distress
- For malaria, prophylaxis should be started 2 weeks before exposure and continue for 4–6 weeks after leaving exposure area
- Rx

QUININE SULFATE
(<u>kwye</u>-nine)

. . . .

METRONIDAZOLE
(meh-troe-<u>nye</u>-da-zole)

(Flagyl, Flagyl ER)

SIDE EFFECTS

Eye disturbances   Anorexia
Nausea, vomiting

NURSING CONSIDERATIONS

- Treatment of malaria, nocturnal leg cramps
- Peak 1–3 hours
- Take at the same time each day to maintain blood level
- Avoid OTC cold meds, tonic water
- May increase digoxin levels
- OTC, Rx

• •

SIDE EFFECTS

Headache   Abdominal cramps
Dizziness   Metallic taste
Nausea, vomiting, diarrhea

NURSING CONSIDERATIONS

- Treatment of a wide variety of infections, including trichomoniasis and giardiasis
- IV: immediate onset, PO: peak 1–2 hours
- Urine may turn dark reddish-brown
- Avoid hazardous activities
- Treatment of both partners is necessary in trichomoniasis
- Do not drink alcohol or preparations containing alcohol during and 48 hours after use, disulfiram-like reaction can occur
- Rx

ISONIAZID
(eye-soe-<u>nye</u>-a-zid)

(INH)

· ·

ACYCLOVIR
(ay-<u>sye</u>-kloe-veer)

(Zovirax)

SIDE EFFECTS

Peripheral neuropathy   Liver damage

NURSING CONSIDERATIONS

- Prevention and treatment of TB
- PO/IM: onset rapid, peak 1–2 hours, duration up to 24 hours
- Contact clinician if signs of hepatitis: yellow eyes and skin, nausea, vomiting, anorexia, dark urine, unusual tiredness, or weakness
- Contact clinician if signs of peripheral neuropathy: numbness, tingling, or weakness
- Monitor liver tests
- Rx

• •

SIDE EFFECTS

Headache   Nausea, vomiting, diarrhea
Blood dyscrasias

NURSING CONSIDERATIONS

- Treatment of herpes, varicella
- IV: onset immediate, peak immediate
- PO: absorbed minimally, onset unknown, peak 90 minutes
- Do not break, crush, or chew capsules
- PO: take without regard to meals with a full glass of water
- If dose is missed, take as soon as remembered, up to 1 hour before next dose
- Contact clinician if sore throat, fever, and fatigue; could be signs of superinfection
- May cause acute renal failure; monitor renal function
- Thrombocytopenic purpura
- Rx

OSELTAMIVIR PHOSPHATE
(oss-el-<u>tam</u>-i-veer)

(Tamiflu)

• •

VALACYCLOVIR HCL
(val-ay-<u>sye</u>-kloe-veer)

(Valtrex)

SIDE EFFECTS

Nausea	Headache
Vomiting	Fatigue
Dizziness	Cough

NURSING CONSIDERATIONS

- Used as prophylaxis in adults for influenza, including avian bird flu
- Used to treat uncomplicated acute flu symptoms in patients that are symptomatic for 2 days or less
- Should not be used as a substitute for influenza vaccinations
- May be taken without regard to meals
- Rx

• •

SIDE EFFECTS

Nausea, vomiting, diarrhea	Rash
Abdominal cramps	Fatigue
Headache	Dizziness

NURSING CONSIDERATIONS

- For the treatment of genital herpes
- Used to treat herpes zoster (shingles)
- Used to treat herpes labialis (cold sores)
- Patients should drink plenty of fluids during treatment
- Avoid sexual contact when lesions are visible
- Use with caution in pregnancy and nursing mothers
- Rx

ZIDOVUDINE
(zye-<u>doe</u>-vyoo-deen)

(AZT, Retrovir)

- -

CEPHALEXIN
(sef-a-<u>lex</u>-in)

(Keflex)

SIDE EFFECTS

Fever, headache, malaise

Nausea, vomiting, diarrhea

Dizziness

Insomnia

Dyspepsia

Anorexia

Rash

NURSING CONSIDERATIONS

- Management of HIV infections and prevention of HIV following needlestick
- GI upset and insomnia resolve after 3–4 weeks
- PO: peak 30–90 minutes
- Rx

• •

SIDE EFFECTS

Diarrhea

Anaphylaxis

Nausea

Rash

Headache

NURSING CONSIDERATIONS

- Treatment of upper and lower respiratory tract, urinary tract, and skin infections, bone infections, otitis media Peak 1 hour, duration usually 6 hours, but may be up to 12 hours with decreased renal function
- Take for 10–14 days to prevent superinfection
- Possible cross-allergy to penicillin
- May cause false positive of urine glucose
- Rx

CEFUROXIME

(sef-yoor-<u>ox</u>-eem)

(Ceftin, Zinacef)

• •

CEFDINIR

(<u>sef</u>-di-neer)

(Omnicef)

SIDE EFFECTS

Diarrhea   Rash

NURSING CONSIDERATIONS

- Treatment of respiratory tract, urinary tract, bone and skin infections, gonococcal infections, meningitis, septicemia
- Take for 10–14 days to prevent superinfection
- May cause increased BUN and serum creatine
- May cause false positive urine glucose
- Rx

• •

SIDE EFFECTS

Nausea, vomiting, diarrhea   Headache
Anorexia   Vaginal yeast infection
Rash

NURSING CONSIDERATIONS

- Treatment of acute exacerbations of chronic bronchitis, sinusitis, pharyngitis, otitis media, tonsillitis, skin infections
- Take for 10–14 days to prevent superinfection
- Do not give antacids or iron supplements within 2 hours
- May cause false positive for urine ketones or glucose
- May cause increased GGT
- Rx

CEFEPIME
(<u>sef</u>-e-peem)

(Maxipime)

· ·

CIPROFLOXACIN
(sip-roe-<u>flocks</u>-a-sin)

(Cipro)

SIDE EFFECTS

Nausea, vomiting, diarrhea   Rash
Anorexia   Headache
Elevated liver function tests

NURSING CONSIDERATIONS

- Treatment of respiratory tract, urinary, and skin infections
- IV: peak 30 minutes
- IM: peak 2 hours
- May cause false positive Coombs test
- May cause false positive for urine glucose
- Rx

• •

SIDE EFFECTS

Seizures   Photosensitivity
Nausea, vomiting, diarrhea, abd.   Tendon rupture, muscle tear
  distress, flatulence   CNS side effects
Rash

NURSING CONSIDERATIONS

- Treatment of infection caused by E. coli and other bacteria, chronic bacterial prostatitis, acute sinusitis, postexposure inhalation anthrax
- Contraindicated in children less than 18 years of age
- Take 2 hours pc or 2 hours before an antacid or iron preparation
- Take at equal intervals around the clock
- Avoid caffeine
- Encourage fluids to 8–10 glasses/day
- May cause false positive in opiate screening tests
- Do not infuse with other medications
- Rx

LEVOFLOXACIN
(lee-voe-<u>flocks</u>-a-sin)

(Levaquin)

· ·

Anti-Infectives
Glycopeptides

VANCOMYCIN
(van-koe-<u>my</u>-sin)

(Vancocin)

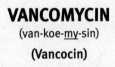

SIDE EFFECTS

Headache, nausea, vomiting, diarrhea, constipation
Stomach pain
Dizziness, heartburn
Vaginal itching and/or discharge
Tendon rupture or tendinitis

Irritation, pain, tenderness, redness, warmth, or swelling at the injection spot
Seizures, confusion, rash
Hallucination, paranoia
Angioedema

NURSING CONSIDERATIONS

- Treatment of infections such as endocarditis, tuberculosis, anthrax, pneumonia, chronic bronchitis, and infections involving the sinus, urinary tract, kidney, prostate, or skin
- Infused injection over 60–90 minutes, once every 24 hours
- Teach patient to avoid sunlamps and tanning beds and to limit time in sun
- Avoid activities that require alertness or coordination
- Monitor for hepatotoxicity
- May increase risk of suicidal thoughts or behaviors
- Monitor blood sugar; may cause hypoglycemia or hyperglycemia
- Teach patient to notify physician immediately for change in heartbeat
- Rx

• •

SIDE EFFECTS

Liver damage
Nephrotoxicity

Tinnitus or hearing loss

NURSING CONSIDERATIONS

- Treatment of resistant staph infections, colitis, staph enterocolitis, endocarditis prophylaxis for dental procedures (used for *C. difficile*)
- PO: poor absorption
- IV: peak 5 minutes, duration 12–24 hours
- Give at least 60 minutes (IV); do not infuse with other drugs
- Give antihistamine if "red man syndrome": decreased blood pressure, flushing of face and neck
- Contact clinician if signs of superinfection: sore throat, fever, fatigue
- Rx

CLINDAMYCIN HCL PHOSPHATE
(<u>klin</u>-da-my-sin)

(Cleocin HCL, Cleocin Phosphate for IM)

• •

AZITHROMYCIN
(a-zi-thro-<u>my</u>-sin)

(Zithromax)

SIDE EFFECTS

Nausea, vomiting, diarrhea   Rash
Abdominal pain   Jaundice
Vaginitis

NURSING CONSIDERATIONS

- Treatment of infections caused by Staphylococcus, Streptococcus, and other organisms
- PO: peak 45 minutes, duration 6 hours
- IM: peak 3 hours, duration 8–12 hours
- May cause increase in AST, ALT, CPK
- Rx

● ●

SIDE EFFECTS

Nausea, vomiting, diarrhea

NURSING CONSIDERATIONS

- Treatment of mild to moderate infections of the respiratory tract, skin, nongonococcal urethritis, cervicitis, acute pharyngitis/tonsillitis, community acquired pneumonia
- PO: rapid onset, peak 2.5–3.2 hours, duration 24 hours
- IV: rapid onset, peak end of infusion, duration 24 hours
- PO: don't take with antacids; can take with or without food
- Monitor for signs of superinfection (diarrhea, perineal itching, oral ulcers)
- If treated for nongonococcal urethritis or cervicitis, sexual partners also need treatment
- Rx

CLARITHROMYCIN

(kla-<u>rith</u>-row-my-sin)

(Biaxin, Biaxin XL)

• •

ERYTHROMYCIN

(eh-rith-roe-<u>my</u>-sin)

(Ery-Tab, Erythrocin)

SIDE EFFECTS

Nausea

Taste abnormalities

Diarrhea

Dyspepsia

Headache

NURSING CONSIDERATIONS

- Used for respiratory infections, pharyngitis/tonsillitis, sinusitis
- Treatment may be 7–14 days depending on organism and extent of infection
- Medication should be taken with food
- Be aware of possible increase in theophylline and carbamazepine levels
- Rx

• •

SIDE EFFECTS

Abdominal cramps

Pain at injection site

Nausea, vomiting, diarrhea

Rash

Anaphylaxis

NURSING CONSIDERATIONS

- Treatment of infections, including chlamydia, syphilis
- PO: give 1 hr ac/2 hr pc with full glass water (avoid citrus juice); some formulations can be given without regard to meals
- PO: onset 1 hour, peak up to 4 hours, duration 6–12 hours
- IV: onset rapid, peak end of infusion, duration 6–12 hours
- Take at equal intervals around the clock
- Can be used in patients with compromised renal function
- Monitor for signs of superinfection (diarrhea, perineal itching, oral ulcers)
- Rx

AMOXICILLIN, AMPICILLIN, PENICILLIN

(ah-mox-i-<u>sill</u>-in, am-pi-<u>sill</u>-in, pen-i-<u>sill</u>-in)

(Bicillin, Omnipen, Wycillin)

. . . .

TRIMETHOPRIM/ SULFAMETHOXAZOLE

(trye-<u>meth</u>-oh-prim sul-fa-meth-<u>ox</u>-a-zole)

(Bactrim, Septra)

SIDE EFFECTS

Allergic reactions: fever, difficulty breathing, skin rash
Renal, hepatic, hematologic abnormalities

Nausea, vomiting, diarrhea

NURSING CONSIDERATIONS

- Treatment of respiratory infections, scarlet fever, otitis media, pneumonia, skin and soft tissue infections, gonorrhea
- Take careful history of penicillin reaction; observe for 20 minutes post IM injection
- PO for penicillin and ampicillin: take 1 hr ac or 2 hr pc to reduce gastric acid destruction of drug; not true for amoxicillin
- Take equally divided doses around the clock
- Continue medication for entire time prescribed, even if symptoms resolve
- Check for hypersensitivity to other drugs, especially cephalosporins
- Rx

• •

SIDE EFFECTS

Hypersensitivity reaction
Blood dyscrasias
Photosensitivity

Nausea, vomiting, anorexia
Stomatitis, abdominal pain

NURSING CONSIDERATIONS

- Treatment of UTI, chancroid, acute otitis media, acute and chronic prostatitis, shigellosis, pneumonitis, chronic bronchitis, traveler's diarrhea
- PO: with full glass water; if upset stomach occurs, take with food
- PO: take at equal intervals around the clock
- IV solution must be given slowly over 60–90 minutes; flush lines at end of infusion to remove residue
- Monitor for hypersensitivity reaction; stop med at first sign of skin rash
- Never administer IM, rapidly IV, or by bolus injection
- Encourage fluids to 8–10 glasses/day
- Rx

DOXYCYCLINE HYCLATE
(dox-i-<u>sye</u>-kleen <u>hye</u>-klate)
(Vibramycin, Vibra-Tabs)

• •

MINOCYCLINE HCL
(mi-noe-<u>sye</u>-kleen)
(Minocin)

SIDE EFFECTS

Photosensitivity
GI upset, diarrhea
Renal, hepatic, hematologic
  abnormalities

Dental discoloration of
  deciduous (baby) teeth

NURSING CONSIDERATIONS

- Treatment of syphilis, chlamydia, gonorrhea, chronic periodontitis, acne, anthrax; malaria prophylaxis
- Peak 1.5–4 hours
- If GI symptoms occur, administer with food EXCEPT milk products or other foods high in calcium (interferes with absorption)
- Take with full glass of water; do NOT take within 1 hour of bedtime or reclining
- Check patient's tongue for monilial infection
- Discard outdated prescriptions
- Avoid prolonged exposure to direct sunlight or UV light
- Avoid during tooth and early development periods (4th month prenatal to 8 years of age)
- Anticoagulant therapy may need to be adjusted
- Rx

• •

SIDE EFFECTS

Photosensitivity
GI upset, diarrhea
Renal, hepatic, hematologic
  abnormalities

Dental discoloration of
  deciduous (baby) teeth

NURSING CONSIDERATIONS

- Treatment of chlamydia, periodontitis, acne, Rocky Mountain spotted fever, respiratory tract infections, meningitis
- Peak 2–3 hours
- If GI symptoms occur, administer with food EXCEPT milk products or other foods high in calcium (interferes with absorption)
- Take with full glass of water; do NOT take within 1 hour of bedtime
- Check patient's tongue for monilial infection
- Discard outdated prescriptions
- Avoid prolonged exposure to direct sunlight or UV light
- Avoid during tooth and early development periods (4th month prenatal to 8 years of age)
- Rx

HYDROCORTISONE
(hye-dro-<u>kor</u>-ti-sone)

(Cortef, Solu-Cortef)

· ·

METHYLPREDNISOLONE
(meth-ill-pred-<u>niss</u>-oh-lone)

(Medrol)

SIDE EFFECTS

Depression
Flushing, sweating
Hypertension

Nausea, diarrhea
Hyperglycemia
Psychic derangements

NURSING CONSIDERATIONS

- Treatment of severe inflammation, septic shock, adrenal insufficiency, ulcerative colitis, collagen disorders
- Med masks signs of infection, so check for elevated temperature, WBC count
- PO: take with food, milk, antacids
- IM: give deep into gluteal UOQ, avoid deltoid, rotate sites, avoid subQ administration because it may damage tissue
- Monitor blood sugar in diabetes carefully
- Rectal: for colitis, retain med for 20 minutes, onset 3–5 days
- Wear medical information tag
- Do not mix with other medicines
- Rx

• •

SIDE EFFECTS

Peptic ulcer/possible perforation
Hypertension and circulatory
  problems

Poor wound healing
Hyperglycemia
Psychic derangements

NURSING CONSIDERATIONS

- Treatment of severe inflammation, shock, adrenal insufficiency, management of acute spinal cord injury, collagen disorders
- PO: take with food, milk, antacids
- PO: peak 1–2 hours, duration 1.5 days
- IM: give deep into gluteal UOQ, avoid deltoid, rotate sites, avoid subQ administration because it may damage tissue
- IM: peak 4–8 days, duration 1–4 weeks
- Eat food high in protein, calcium, vitamin D; avoid sodium
- Contact clinician if anorexia, difficulty breathing, weakness, dizziness; symptoms may appear during periods of stress or trauma
- Contact clinician if black/tarry stools, slow wound healing, blurred vision, bruising/bleeding, weight gain, emotional changes
- Wear medical information tag
- Monitor patient weight, blood sugars
- Rx

PREDNISOLONE
(pred-<u>niss</u>-oh-lone)

(Delta-Cortef, Flo-Pred, Prelone)

· ·

PREDNISONE
(<u>pred</u>-ni-sone)

(Deltasone, Meticorten)

SIDE EFFECTS

Depression
Hypertension, circulatory
  problems

Nausea, diarrhea
Abdominal distention

NURSING CONSIDERATIONS

- Treatment of severe inflammation, immunosuppression, neoplasms
- PO: take with food, milk, antacids
- PO: peak 1–2 hours, duration 3–36 hours
- IM: give deep into gluteal UOQ, avoid deltoid, rotate sites, avoid subQ administration because it may damage tissue
- IM: peak 1 hour, duration 4 weeks
- Eat food high in protein, calcium, vitamin D; avoid sodium
- Contact clinician if anorexia, difficulty breathing, weakness, dizziness; symptoms may appear during periods of stress or trauma
- Contact clinician if black/tarry stools, slow wound healing, blurred vision, bruising/bleeding, weight gain, emotional changes
- Wear medical information tag
- Rx

· ·

SIDE EFFECTS

Peptic ulcer/possible perforation
Depression
Hypertension, circulatory
  problems

Nausea, diarrhea
Abdominal distention
Hyperglycemia
Psychic derangements

NURSING CONSIDERATIONS

- Treatment of severe inflammation, immune suppression, neoplasms, multiple sclerosis, collagen disorders, dermatologic disorders, myasthenia gravis
- PO: take with food, milk, antacids
- PO: peak 1–2 hours, duration 24–36 hours
- Eat food high in protein, calcium, vitamin D; avoid sodium
- Contact clinician if anorexia, difficulty breathing, weakness, dizziness; symptoms may appear during periods of stress or trauma
- Contact clinician if black/tarry stools, slow wound healing, blurred vision, bruising/bleeding, weight gain, emotional changes
- Excessive consumption of licorice can increase risk of hypokalemia
- Wear medical information tag
- Monitor blood sugar in diabetic patients
- Rx

Anti-Inflammatory Medications
Nonsteroidal Anti-Inflammatories

NABUMETONE
(na-<u>byoo</u>-meh-tone)

• •

Anti-Inflammatory Medications
Nonsteroidal Anti-Inflammatories

IBUPROFEN
(eye-byoo-<u>proe</u>-fen)

(Advil, Motrin IB)

SIDE EFFECTS

Abdominal pain	Flatulence	Headache
Constipation	Tinnitus	Rash
Diarrhea	Edema	Gastritis

NURSING CONSIDERATIONS

- Used to manage symptoms of osteoarthritis and rheumatoid arthritis
- Take with food or milk
- Contraindicated in patients with hypersensitivity to other NSAIDs
- Alcohol may increase ulcerogenic effects if used concurrently
- May take 2 weeks or more to notice improvement
- Rx

• •

SIDE EFFECTS

Headache	Blood dyscrasias	Rash
Nausea, anorexia	Hives	
GI bleeding	Facial swelling	

NURSING CONSIDERATIONS

- Treatment of rheumatoid arthritis, osteoarthritis, primary dysmenorrhea, gout, dental pain, musculoskeletal disorders, fever, headache, menstrual cramps
- Onset: 30 minutes, peak 1–2 hours
- Full therapeutic effect may take up to 1 month
- Contact clinician if blurred vision, ringing or roaring in ears, which may indicate toxicity
- Contact clinician if changes in urinary pattern, increased weight, edema, increased pain in joints, fever, blood in urine, which may indicate kidney damage
- Avoid use with ASA, NSAIDs, and alcohol, which may precipitate GI bleeding
- Take with food or milk
- Possible cross-allergy with aspirin
- OTC, Rx

Anti-Inflammatory Medications
Nonsteroidal Anti-Inflammatories

NAPROXEN
(na-<u>prox</u>-en)

(Aleve [OTC], Anaprox, Naprosyn)

• •

Antineoplastics
Antineoplastics

METHOTREXATE
(meth-oh-<u>trex</u>-ate)

(Trexall)

SIDE EFFECTS

GI bleeding
Blood dyscrasias
Hives
Rash
Asthma

NURSING CONSIDERATIONS

- Management of mild to moderate pain; treatment of rheumatoid, juvenile, and gouty arthritis, osteoarthritis, primary dysmenorrhea
- Patients with asthma, ASA hypersensitivity, or nasal polyps have increased risk of hypersensitivity
- Contact clinician if blurred vision, ringing or roaring in ears, which may indicate toxicity
- Contact clinician if black stools, flulike symptoms
- Contact clinician if changes in urinary pattern, increased weight, edema, increased pain in joints, fever, blood in urine, which may indicate kidney damage
- Use sunscreen to prevent photosensitivity
- Avoid use with ASA, steroids, and alcohol
- OTC, Rx

• •

SIDE EFFECTS

Nausea, vomiting, diarrhea   Ulcerative stomatitis
Anorexia   Dizziness
Alopecia

NURSING CONSIDERATIONS

- Treatment of cancer, mycosis fungoides, psoriasis, rheumatoid arthritis
- PO, IM, IV: onset 4–7 days, peak 7–14 days, duration 21 days
- Avoid crowds and people with known infections
- Do not take with ASA or other NSAIDs, which may cause GI bleeding
- Monitor for pulmonary toxicity, which may manifest early as a dry, nonproductive cough
- Rx

TAMOXIFEN
(ta-<u>mox</u>-i-fen)

· ·

Cardiovascular Medications
ACE Inhibitors

BENAZEPRIL HCL
(ben-<u>ay</u>-ze-pril)

(Lotensin)

SIDE EFFECTS

Nausea, vomiting
Hot flashes
Rash
Vaginal discharge

Irregular menses
Fluid retention
Depression, mood disturbances

NURSING CONSIDERATIONS

- Management of advanced breast cancer not responsive to other therapy in estrogen-receptor-positive patients
- Peak 4–7 hours
- To decrease GI upset, take after antacid, after evening meal, before bedtime, or take antiemetic 30–60 minutes ahead
- Vaginal bleeding, pruritus, hot flashes are reversible after stopping med
- Contact clinician if decreased visual acuity, which may be irreversible
- Tumor flare (increase in tumor size and increased bone pain) may occur, but will decrease rapidly; may take analgesics for pain
- Rx

• •

SIDE EFFECTS

Angioedema
Cough
Headache

Dizziness
Fatigue

NURSING CONSIDERATIONS

- Used to treat hypertension
- Often used in combination with thiazide diuretics
- Indomethacin may decrease therapeutic effects
- Avoid salt substitutes containing potassium because of potassium-sparing effect
- Avoid nonprescription cough medications unless physician directed
- Rx

CAPTOPRIL

(<u>kap</u>-toe-pril)

(Capoten)

• •

ENALAPRIL

(e-<u>nal</u>-a-pril)

(Vasotec)

SIDE EFFECTS

Bronchospasm, dyspnea, cough
Orthostatic hypotension
Dizziness

Tachycardia
Loss of taste

NURSING CONSIDERATIONS

- Treatment of hypertension, CHF, left ventricular dysfunction after MI, diabetic neuropathy
- Contact clinician if fever, skin rash, sore throat, mouth sores, swelling of hands or feet, fast or irregular heartbeat, chest pain, or cough
- Take on empty stomach 1 hour before meals or 2 hours after; tablets may be crushed and mixed with juice or soft food for ease of swallowing
- Loss of taste might last for first 2–3 months, clinical concern is interference with nutrition
- Avoid changing positions (sitting/standing/lying) rapidly, esp. during the first few days before body adjusts to med
- Do not use OTC (cough, cold, or allergy) meds unless directed by clinician
- Avoid potassium supplements and potassium salt substitute
- Rx

• •

SIDE EFFECTS

Headache
Dizziness, hypotension
Tachycardia
Tinnitus

Hyperkalemia
Angioedema
Persistent cough

NURSING CONSIDERATIONS

- Treatment of hypertension, CHF, left ventricular dysfunction
- Contact clinician if fever, skin rash, sore throat, mouth sores, swelling of hands or feet, fast or irregular heartbeat, chest pain, or cough
- Avoid changing positions (sitting/standing/lying) rapidly, esp. during the first few days before body adjusts to med
- Cardiovascular adverse reactions may reoccur
- Do not use OTC (cough, cold, or allergy) meds unless directed by clinician
- Avoid potassium supplements and potassium salt substitutes
- Rx

LISINOPRIL
(lye-<u>sin</u>-oh-pril)

(Prinivil, Zestril)

• •

RAMIPRIL
(<u>ram</u>-ih-pril)

(Altace)

SIDE EFFECTS

Headache	Tachycardia
Dizziness	Fatigue
Nausea, vomiting, diarrhea	SIADH
Hypotension	Cough

NURSING CONSIDERATIONS

- Treatment of mild to moderate hypertension, systolic CHF, acute MI
- Avoid changing positions (lying/sitting/standing) rapidly
- May take without regard to food
- Avoid high-sodium foods (canned soups, lunch meats, cheese)
- Avoid high-potassium foods (bananas, citrus fruits, raisins)
- Rx

• •

SIDE EFFECTS

Headache	Nausea
Hypotension	Cough
Dizziness	Fatigue
Vertigo	

NURSING CONSIDERATIONS

- Treatment of hypertension, CHF following MI, reduce risk of death from CV causes in patients with risk factors
- Can mix capsule contents with water, juice, or applesauce to aid swallowing
- Avoid changing positions (lying/sitting/standing) rapidly
- Contact clinician if persistent, dry, nonproductive cough; increased SOB; edema; or unusual bruising or bleeding
- Avoid salt substitutes containing potassium
- Rx

DOXAZOSIN MESYLATE
(dox-<u>ay</u>-zoe-sin)

(Cardura)

• •

PRAZOSIN HCL
(<u>pray</u>-zoh-sin)

(Minipress)

SIDE EFFECTS

Dizziness	Fatigue, malaise
Headache	Priapism (rare)

NURSING CONSIDERATIONS

- Treatment of hypertension, benign prostatic hyperplasia (BPH)
- Avoid changing positions (lying/sitting/standing) rapidly
- Can have first-dose syncope, maintain recumbent for 90 minutes
- Full therapeutic effects may require several weeks of therapy
- Avoid high-sodium foods (canned soups, lunch meats, cheese)
- Use caution in potentially hazardous activities until stabilized
- Avoid alcohol, smoking
- Wear medical information tag
- Rx

• •

SIDE EFFECTS

Dizziness	Headache
Nausea, vomiting, diarrhea	Palpitations
Drowsiness	Syncope

NURSING CONSIDERATIONS

- Treatment of hypertension
- Onset 2 hours, peak 1–3 hours, duration 6–12 hours
- Can have first-dose syncope, take the first dose (and any increment) at bedtime, do not drive for 24 hours
- Full therapeutic effects may require 4–6 weeks of therapy
- Food may delay absorption
- Avoid changing positions (lying/sitting/standing) rapidly
- Check with clinician before using OTC cold, cough, and allergy meds
- Rx

Cardiovascular Medications
Alpha Blockers

TERAZOSIN HCL
(ter-<u>ay</u>-zoh-sin)

(Hytrin)

· ·

Cardiovascular Medications
Angiotensin Receptor Blockers

VALSARTAN
(val-<u>sar</u>-tan)

(Diovan)

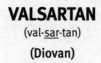

SIDE EFFECTS

Dizziness	Nausea
Headache	Weakness
Drowsiness	Syncope

NURSING CONSIDERATIONS

- Treatment of hypertension, BPH
- Avoid changing positions (lying/sitting/standing) rapidly
- Can have first-dose syncope, take the first dose (and any increment) at bedtime; do not drive or operate machinery for 4 hours
- Rx

• •

SIDE EFFECTS

Headache	Nausea, vomiting, diarrhea	High blood creatinine
Dizziness	Hypotension	Rash
Excessive tiredness; fatigue	Viral infection	Vasculitis
Stomach, back, or joint pain	Cough, flu symptoms	

NURSING CONSIDERATIONS

- Treatment of hypertension; treatment of CHF in patients who cannot take an ACE inhibitor; reduction of cardiovascular mortality in patients with left ventricular failure or left ventricular dysfunction after MI
- Take once daily for high blood pressure; twice daily for CHF
- Avoid salt substitutes containing potassium
- Monitor blood creatine; may decrease kidney function
- May have cross-allergy to sulfonamides
- Rx

VALSARTAN
HYDROCHLOROTHIAZIDE
(val-<u>sar</u>-tan hye-droe-klor-oh-<u>thye</u>-a-zide)

(Diovan HCT)

• •

Cardiovascular Medications
Antianginals

ISOSORBIDE DINITRATE
(eye-soe-<u>sor</u>-bide)

(Isordil)

SIDE EFFECTS

Headache
Dizziness
Excessive tiredness; fatigue
Stomach, back, or joint pain
Nausea, vomiting, diarrhea

Hypotension
Viral infection
Cough, flu symptoms
High blood creatinine
Rash
Blurred vision

Nasopharyngitis
Tinnitus, vertigo
GI distress
Male sexual dysfunction

NURSING CONSIDERATIONS

- Treatment of hypertension; treatment of CHF in patients who cannot take an ACE inhibitor
- Take once daily for high blood pressure; twice daily for CHF
- Avoid salt substitutes containing potassium
- Monitor blood sugars in diabetic patients; may cause hyperglycemia
- NSAIDs may reduce the effect of diuretic
- May cause exacerbation of SLE
- May have cross-allergy to sulfonamides
- Rx

. . . .

SIDE EFFECTS

Dizziness, postural hypotension
Vascular headache, flushing
Drowsiness

Nausea
Lightheadedness

NURSING CONSIDERATIONS

- Treatment/prophylaxis of angina pectoris, CHF
- PO: 1 hour before food or 2 hours after meals for maximum absorption, but taking with food may reduce or eliminate headache
- Chewable tablet: chew well, hold in mouth for 2 minutes before swallowing
- Sublingual: dissolve under tongue; do not eat, drink, talk or smoke during use; go to ED if pain not relieved in 15 minutes
- Avoid changing positions (lying/sitting/standing) rapidly
- Use caution in potentially hazardous activities until stabilized
- Avoid alcohol, smoking, strenuous exercise in hot environment
- Wear medical information tag
- Rx

ISOSORBIDE MONONITRATE
(eye-soe-<u>sor</u>-bide)

(Ismo)

• •

NITROGLYCERIN
(nye-troe-<u>gli</u>-ser-in)

(Nitro-Par, Transderm-Nitro/Nitrostat)

SIDE EFFECTS

Dizziness, postural hypotension   Drowsiness
Vascular headache, flushing   Nausea

NURSING CONSIDERATIONS

- Treatment/prophylaxis of angina pectoris
- PO: 1 hour before food or 2 hours after meals for maximum absorption, but taking with food may reduce or eliminate headache
- Chewable tablet: chew well, hold in mouth for 2 minutes before swallowing
- Sublingual: dissolve under tongue; do not eat, drink, talk, or smoke during use; go to ED if pain not relieved in 15 minutes
- Avoid changing positions (lying/sitting/standing) rapidly
- Use caution in potentially hazardous activities until stabilized
- Avoid alcohol, smoking, strenuous exercise in hot environment
- Wear medical information tag
- Rx

• •

SIDE EFFECTS

Transient headache   Flushing
Postural hypotension

NURSING CONSIDERATIONS

- Treatment/prophylaxis of angina pectoris; IV used for control of BP during surgery and CHF associated with acute MI
- Sustained-release: take every 6–12 hours on an empty stomach; onset 20–45 minutes, duration 3–8 hours
- Sublingual: patient sitting/lying should let tablet dissolve under tongue and not swallow saliva; onset 1–3 minutes, duration 30 minutes
- Spray: hold canister vertically, spray on tongue, close mouth immediately, do not inhale spray; onset 2 minutes, duration 30–60 minutes
- IV: use infusion pump and special non-PVC tubing; onset 1–2 minutes, duration 3–5 minutes
- Ointment: spread on skin in thin uniform layer; onset 30–60 minutes, duration 2–12 hours
- Transdermal: apply to clean hairless area; rotate sites; onset 30–60 minutes, duration 12–24 hours
- Go to ED if pain not relieved with 3 tablets in 15 minutes
- Wear medical information tag
- Rx

AMIODARONE HCL
(am-ee-<u>oh</u>-da-rone)

(Cordarone, Pacerone)

• •

Cardiovascular Medications
Antiarrhythmics

LIDOCAINE HCL
(<u>lye</u>-doe-kane)

(Xylocaine)

SIDE EFFECTS

Dizziness, fatigue, malaise
Corneal microdeposits
Bradycardia, hypotension
Anorexia, constipation
Photosensitivity

Neurologic dysfunction
Muscle weakness
Cardiac arrest
Nausea, vomiting

NURSING CONSIDERATIONS

- Management of ventricular arrhythmias unresponsive to less toxic agents
- IV: continuous cardiac monitoring
- Assess for signs of pulmonary toxicity: rales/crackles, decreased breath sounds, pleuritic friction rub, fatigue, dyspnea, cough, pleuritic pain, fever
- Neurotoxicity (ataxia, muscle weakness, tingling or numbness in fingers or toes, uncontrolled movements, tremors) common during initial therapy
- Side effects may not appear until several days, weeks, or years and may persist for several months after stopping med
- Teach patient to check radial pulse
- Use sunscreen and protective clothing to prevent photosensitivity
- May increase ALT, AST
- Rx

• •

SIDE EFFECTS

Hypotension, tremors
Double vision
Tinnitus
Respiratory depression/arrest
Confusion, blurred vision

Drowsiness, dizziness
Twitching, convulsions
Bradycardia
Visual color disturbances

NURSING CONSIDERATIONS

- Used for premature ventricular contractions
- Give oxygen; have resuscitation equipment available
- IV: use infusion pump; patient on cardiac monitor
- Check BUN, creatinine
- Monitor lungs for rales
- Rx

PROCAINAMIDE
(proe-<u>kane</u>-a-mide)

• •

QUINIDINE
(<u>kwin</u>-i-deen)

SIDE EFFECTS

Hypotension	Fever, rash	Anxiety
Bradycardia	Dizziness	
Nausea, vomiting	Neutropenia	

NURSING CONSIDERATIONS

- Management of life-threatening ventricular dysrhythmias and maintain NSR following conversion of atrial arrhythmia
- IV: use infusion pump; monitor BP every 5–15 minutes; on cardiac monitor; keep patient recumbent
- IV: monitor CBC, blood levels, I & O, daily weight
- PO: best absorption on empty stomach, may take with food to decrease GI upset
- Take at equal intervals around the clock
- Teach patient to check radial pulse
- Avoid caffeine
- May increase alkaline phosphatase, bilirium, lactic dehydrogenase, AST
- Rx

. . . .

SIDE EFFECTS

Anemia	Tinnitus
Hypotension	Fever
Nausea, vomiting, diarrhea	Fatigue
Headache	Vision changes
Heart block	

NURSING CONSIDERATIONS

- Used for atrial or ventricular arrhythmias and to test malaria
- May increase toxicity for digitalis
- Monitor liver function tests and I & O
- Check apical pulse and BP
- Monitor EKG and BP
- Avoid changing positions (lying/sitting/standing) rapidly
- Avoid use with alcohol, caffeine, smoking
- Patient should wear medical information tag
- Rx

SOTALOL
(<u>soe</u>-ta-lole)

(Betapace)

• •

Cardiovascular Medications
Antihypertensives

BISOPROLOL
(bis-<u>oh</u>-pro-lole)

(Zebeta)

SIDE EFFECTS

Fatigue
Weakness
Impotence
Bradycardia

Dyspnea
Life-threatening ventricular
  arrhythmias
Hyperglycemia

NURSING CONSIDERATIONS

- Management of life-threatening ventricular arrhythmias
- Teach patient to check radial pulse; if less than 50, hold med and contact clinician
- Change positions (sitting/standing/lying) slowly
- Avoid activities that require alertness until drug response known
- Contact clinician if slow pulse, difficulty breathing, wheezing, cold hands and feet, dizziness, confusion, depression, rash, fever, sore throat, unusual bleeding or bruising
- Milk products may decrease absorption
- Rx

● ●

SIDE EFFECTS

GI upset
Fatigue
Weakness

Dizziness
Headache

NURSING CONSIDERATIONS

- Treatment of mild to moderate hypertension
- Peak: 2–4 hours
- Therapeutic response in 1–2 weeks
- Do not stop med abruptly; may precipitate angina
- Do not use OTC meds with stimulants, such as nasal deconges-tants or cold meds, unless directed
- Avoid alcohol, smoking, sodium intake
- Contact clinician if signs of CHF: difficulty breathing, night cough, swelling of extremities
- Rx

CLONIDINE PATCH
(<u>kloe</u>-ni-deen)

(Catapres, Catapres TTS oral tablets)

• •

HYDRALAZINE HCL
(hye-<u>dral</u>-a-zeen)

SIDE EFFECTS

Drowsiness, sedation
Severe rebound hypertension
Dry mouth and eyes

Dizziness
Headache
Constipation

NURSING CONSIDERATIONS

- Treatment of hypertension, severe cancer pain (in combination with opiates)
- Avoid changing positions (lying/sitting/standing) rapidly
- Avoid use with alcohol, CNS depressants
- Avoid high-sodium foods (canned soups, lunch meats, cheese)
- Use caution in potentially hazardous activities
- Avoid alcohol, smoking, strenuous exercise in hot environment
- Apply patch to nonhairy area (upper outer arm, anterior chest), rotate sites, do not apply to scarred or irritated area
- Wear medical information tag
- Caution patients who wear contact lens that drug may cause dry eyes
- May cause a positive Coombs test
- Rx

• •

SIDE EFFECTS

Headache
Palpitations, tachycardia, angina
Edema
Lupus erythematosus-like
  syndrome
Anorexia

Tremors
Dizziness
Anxiety
Flushing
Rash
Nausea, vomiting, diarrhea

NURSING CONSIDERATIONS

- Used to treat essential hypertension; also for heart valve replacement and treatment of CHF
- PO: give with meals to enhance absorption
- Observe mental status
- Check for weight gain, edema
- Avoid changing positions (lying/sitting/standing) rapidly
- Contact clinician if chest pain, severe fatigue, fever, muscle, or joint pain
- Do not confuse with hydroxyzine
- Rx

HYDROCHLOROTHIAZIDE/ LISINOPRIL
(hye-droe-klor-oh-<u>thye</u>-a-zide/
lye-<u>sin</u>-oh-pril)

(Prinzide, Zestoretic)

• •

Cardiovascular Medications
Antilipemic Agents

ATORVASTATIN CALCIUM
(a-<u>tor</u>-va-stat-in)

(Lipitor)

SIDE EFFECTS

Headache
Dizziness
Nausea, vomiting, diarrhea
Hypotension
Tachycardia

Fatigue
Cough
Muscle cramps
Angioedema

NURSING CONSIDERATIONS

- Used to treat essential hypertension
- Avoid changing positions (lying/sitting/standing) rapidly
- May take without regard to food
- Avoid high-sodium foods (canned soups, lunch meats, cheese)
- Avoid high-potassium foods (bananas, citrus fruits, raisins)
- Rx

• •

SIDE EFFECTS

Constipation
Decreased vitamins A, D, K
Abdominal pain
Nausea

Arthralgia
Myopathy
Nasopharyngitis
UTI

NURSING CONSIDERATIONS

- Used to lower cholesterol levels; treat digitalis toxicity, biliary obstruction pruritus, and diarrhea; decrease risk of MI and stroke in patient with diabetes type 2
- Take other meds 1 hour before or 4 hours after this med to avoid poor absorption
- Mix granules in applesauce or liquid, do not take dry, let stand for 2 minutes
- Monitor for hypoprothrombinemia: bleeding gums, tarry stools, hematuria, bruising
- Monitor liver enzymes
- Avoid grapefruit products
- Rx

EZETIMIBE
(e-<u>zet</u>-i-mibe)

(Zetia, with simvastatin Vytorin)

FLUVASTATIN
(<u>floo</u>-va-sta-tin)

(Lescol)

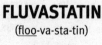

SIDE EFFECTS

Diarrhea   Fatigue
Joint pain

NURSING CONSIDERATIONS

- Used to lower cholesterol
- Ezetimibe is not a statin; can be used with a statin or alone; works by removing cholesterol from the small intestine (statins work in the liver)
- Contact prescriber immediately if unexplained muscle pain, tenderness, or weakness; in rare cases, can cause breakdown of skeletal muscle tissue, leading to kidney failure
- Rx

• •

SIDE EFFECTS

Confusion   Decrease in or urine or
Urinary pain   dark urine
                                  Swelling or weight gain

NURSING CONSIDERATIONS

- Used to lower total cholesterol by preventing formation of cholesterol by the liver
- Contact prescriber immediately if unexplained muscle pain, tenderness, or weakness; in rare cases, can cause breakdown of skeletal muscle tissue, leading to kidney failure
- Rx

LOVASTATIN
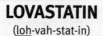
(<u>loh</u>-vah-stat-in)

(Mevacor)

· ·

NIACIN
(<u>nye</u>-a-sin)

**(Niacor for immediate release,
Niaspan for sustained release)**

SIDE EFFECTS

Flatus, constipation
Abdominal pain, nausea, diar-
    rhea, GI upset
Heartburn
Muscle cramps

Dizziness
Headache
Tremor
Blurred vision
Rash, pruritus

NURSING CONSIDERATIONS

- Used to lower cholesterol levels, primary and secondary prevention of coronary events
- Use sunscreen to prevent photosensitivity reactions
- Schedule liver function tests every 1–2 months during the first 1.5 years
- Onset 2 weeks, peak 4–6 weeks, duration 6 weeks
- Take with food, absorption is reduced by 30% on an empty stomach
- Contact clinician if unexplained muscle pain, tenderness or weakness, especially if with fever or malaise
- Rx

• •

SIDE EFFECTS

Headache
Nausea
Postural hypotension
Myopathy

Flushing
Cough
Pruritus

NURSING CONSIDERATIONS

- Treatment of pellagra, hyperlipidemias, peripheral vascular disease
- Take with meals to reduce GI upset, can add 325 mg ASA 30 minutes before dose to reduce flushing
- Flushing will occur several hours after med taken, will decrease over 2 weeks
- Avoid changing positions (sitting/standing/lying) rapidly
- May be used in combination with simvastatin or lovastatin
- Monitor liver enzymes
- May increase glucose level
- OTC, Rx

NICOTINIC ACID
(nih-koh-<u>tin</u>-ick)

(Slo-Niacin, vitamin B)

• •

PRAVASTATIN
(<u>pra</u>-va-sta-tin)

(Pravachol)

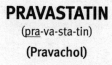

SIDE EFFECTS

Headache
Nausea
Postural hypotension

Flushing
Dry skin

NURSING CONSIDERATIONS

- Treatment of pellagra, hyperlipidemias, peripheral vascular disease
- Take with meals to reduce GI upset, can add 325 mg ASA 30 minutes before dose to reduce flushing
- Flushing will occur several hours after med taken, will decrease over 2 weeks
- Avoid changing positions (sitting/standing/lying) rapidly
- Taking NSAIDs may reduce flushing
- May alter blood sugar
- Monitor liver enzymes
- OTC, Rx

• •

SIDE EFFECTS

Abdominal cramps, flatus
Heartburn

Constipation, diarrhea

NURSING CONSIDERATIONS

- Treatment of hypercholesterolemia, apolipoprotein B (apo B), risk reduction of recurrent MI, atherosclerosis
- Schedule liver function tests semiannually
- Take without regard to food
- Contact clinician if unexplained muscle pain, tenderness, or weakness, especially if with fever or malaise
- Rx

ROSUVASTATIN CALCIUM
(roe-sue-vuh-<u>stat</u>-in)

(Crestor)

· ·

SIMVASTATIN
(<u>sim</u>-va-sta-tin)

(Zocor)

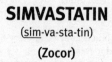

SIDE EFFECTS

Myalgia
Constipation
Abdominal pain

Nausea
Myopathy
Rhabdomyolysis

NURSING CONSIDERATIONS

- Used as adjunct therapy to diet to reduce LDL cholesterol and increase HDL cholesterol; slows progression of atherosclerosis
- Patients should discontinue therapy and notify physician in case of pregnancy
- Use with caution in patients with a history of large alcohol consumption
- Liver function tests are recommended every 12 weeks
- Patient should keep tight control of diet during therapy
- May be used in children 10–17 years of age
- Asian patients may require lower dose to begin therapy
- Do not use with niacin
- Rx

• •

SIDE EFFECTS

Eye lens opacities
Liver dysfunction
URI
Headache

Abdominal pain
Constipation
Nausea

NURSING CONSIDERATIONS

- Treatment of hypercholesterolemia, hypertriglyceridemia, hyperlipoproteinemias, coronary artery disease
- Have eye exam before, 1 month after, and then annually after starting med
- Schedule liver function tests semiannually
- Take without regard to food
- Contact clinician if unexplained muscle pain, tenderness or weakness, especially with fever or malaise
- Asian patients should not take niacin while taking simvastatin
- Rx

ATENOLOL

(a-<u>ten</u>-oh-lole)

(Tenormin, with chlorthalidone Tenoretic)

• •

CARVEDILOL

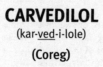

(kar-<u>ved</u>-i-lole)

(Coreg)

SIDE EFFECTS

Bradycardia, cold extremities
Postural hypotension
Bronchospasm in overdose
2nd- or 3rd-degree heart block
Cold extremities

Insomnia, fatigue
Dizziness
Mental changes
Nausea, diarrhea
CHF

NURSING CONSIDERATIONS

- Used in treatment of hypertension, MI, prophylaxis of angina
- Masks signs of hypoglycemia in diabetics
- Teach patient how to take radial pulse
- Check pulse, if less than 50 beats per minute, hold the med and contact clinician
- PO: take before meals, at bedtime
- Tablet may be crushed or swallowed whole
- Do not stop abruptly; taper over 2 weeks
- Rx

• •

SIDE EFFECTS

Dizziness
Diarrhea
Postural hypotension
Impotence
Hyperglycemia

Fatigue
CHF worsening
Dry eyes
Bradycardia

NURSING CONSIDERATIONS

- Used in treatment of hypertension, CHF, LV dysfunction after MI
- PO: take with food
- Tablet may be crushed or swallowed whole
- Do not stop abruptly; taper over 1–2 weeks
- May mask symptoms of low blood sugar in diabetes
- May mask symptoms of hyperthyroidism
- Rx

METOPROLOL SUCCINATE

(meh-<u>toe</u>-proe-lole <u>suk</u>-si-nate)

(Toprol XL, the sustained-release form)

• •

METOPROLOL TARTRATE

(meh-<u>toe</u>-proe-lole)

(Lopressor, the immediate-release form)

SIDE EFFECTS

Bradycardia, palpitations
Nausea, vomiting, diarrhea
Hypotension
CHF

Depression
Insomnia
Dizziness
Confusion

NURSING CONSIDERATIONS

- Used in treatment of hypertension, MI (IV use), prophylaxis of angina, heart failure
- Teach patient how to take radial pulse
- Check pulse, if less than 50 beats per minute, hold the med and contact clinician
- PO: may be taken with food
- Tablet must be swallowed whole
- Do not stop abruptly; taper over 2 weeks; may precipitate angina
- Do not use OTC products (nasal decongestants, cold preparations) unless directed by prescriber
- May worsen heart failure
- May worsen hypoglycemia in diabetes
- Report any dyspnea
- Rx

• •

SIDE EFFECTS

Bradycardia, palpitations
Hypotension
CHF
Nausea, vomiting, diarrhea

Depression
Insomnia
Dizziness
Constipation

NURSING CONSIDERATIONS

- Used in treatment of hypertension, MI (IV use), prophylaxis of angina
- Teach patient how to take radial pulse
- Check pulse, if less than 50 beats per minute, hold the med and contact clinician
- PO: take on an empty stomach, before meals, at bedtime
- Tablet may be crushed or swallowed whole
- Do not stop abruptly; taper over 2 weeks; may precipitate angina
- Do not use OTC products (nasal decongestants, cold preparations) unless directed by prescriber
- May mask hypoglycemia in diabetics
- Report any dyspnea
- Rx

PROPRANOLOL HCL
(proe-<u>pran</u>-oh-lole)

(Inderal)

• •

SOTALOL
(<u>soe</u>-ta-lole)

(Betapace)

SIDE EFFECTS

Weakness	Bronchospasm	Depression
Hypotension	Bradycardia	

NURSING CONSIDERATIONS

- Used in treatment of stable angina, hypertension, dysrhythmias, migraine, prophylaxis MI, essential tremor, alcohol withdrawal, atrial fibrillation
- Teach patient how to take radial pulse
- Check pulse, if less than 50 beats per minute, hold the med and contact clinician
- PO: take with full glass of water at the same time each day
- Do not open, chew, crush extended-release capsule
- Do not stop abruptly; taper over 2 weeks; may precipitate life-threatening dysrhythmias
- Do not use aluminum-containing antacid; may decrease absorption
- May cause cardiac failure
- May cause hypoglycemia in diabetics
- May mask hyperthyroidism
- Rx

• •

SIDE EFFECTS

Fatigue	Dyspnea
Weakness	Life-threatening ventricular
Impotence	arrhythmias
Bradycardia	Hyperglycemia

NURSING CONSIDERATIONS

- Management of life-threatening ventricular arrhythmias
- Teach patient to check radial pulse
- Check pulse; if less than 50 beats per minute, hold med and contact clinician
- Change positions (sitting/standing/lying) slowly
- Avoid activities that require alertness until drug response known
- Contact clinician if slow pulse, difficulty breathing, wheezing, cold hands and feet, dizziness, confusion, depression, rash, fever, sore throat, unusual bleeding or bruising
- Milk products may decrease absorption
- Rx

AMLODIPINE BESYLATE
(am-loh-di-peen bes-i-late)

(Norvasc)

• •

DILTIAZEM HCL
(dil-tye-a-zem)

**(Cardizem, Dilacor, Tiazac,
Cardizem CD [once a day])**

SIDE EFFECTS

Flushing
Edema
Headache
Fatigue

Nausea, vomiting
Abdominal pain
Somnolence

NURSING CONSIDERATIONS

- Used to treat hypertension and documented CAD
- Used also to treat vasospastic angina pectoris
- May be taken without regard to meal
- Consult physician before taking nonprescription cough remedies
- Do not store in bathroom
- Rx

• •

SIDE EFFECTS

Hypotension, dizziness
Edema
Nausea, constipation
Rash

Headache
Fatigue, drowsiness
Angioedema
Bradycardia

NURSING CONSIDERATIONS

- Management of angina, hypertension, vasospasm, atrial fibrillation/flutter, paroxysmal supraventricular tachycardia
- Reduces workload of left ventricle, coronary vasodilator
- Monitor blood pressure during dosage adjustments
- PO: take on an empty stomach, with a full glass of water
- Teach patient how to take radial pulse and keep records of pulse rate
- Avoid hazardous activities until stabilized on drug
- Do not crush, chew, or break
- May increase ALT, AST, LDH, CPK, and alkaline phosphatase
- Rx

FELODIPINE
(fe-<u>loe</u>-di-peen)

• •

NIFEDIPINE
(nye-<u>fed</u>-i-peen)

(Adalat CC, Procardia XL)

SIDE EFFECTS

Dysrhythmia
Headache
Fatigue

Edema
Flushing

NURSING CONSIDERATIONS

- Used in treatment of essential hypertension, angina
- Do not adjust dosage at intervals of less than 2 weeks
- PO: take without regard to meals
- Do not open, chew, or crush extended-release capsule
- Do not use OTC products or alcohol unless directed by prescriber; limit caffeine
- May increase ALT
- Rx

· ·

SIDE EFFECTS

Orthostatic
  hypotension
Peripheral edema
Leg cramps

Chest pain
Headache, dizziness
Impotence
Fatigue

Nausea
Rash

NURSING CONSIDERATIONS

- Used in treatment of hypertension, angina
- Avoid changing positions (sitting/standing/lying) rapidly
- PO: take on an empty stomach; onset 20 minutes, peak
  30 minutes to 6 hours, duration 6–8 hours
- PO, extended-release capsule: do not open, chew, crush; can take without regard
  to meals; duration of 24 hours; shell may appear in stools, but is insignificant
- Do not use OTC products or alcohol unless directed by prescriber; limit caffeine
- Monitor BP when used with beta blockers
- May cause CHF when used with beta blockers
- Do not drink grapefruit juice; stop grapefruit juice at least 3 days prior to
  initiating nifedipine therapy
- Do not take with St. John's wort
- Rx

VERAPAMIL HCL
(ver-ap-a-mill)

(Calan, Covera)

• •

DIGOXIN
(di-jox-in)

(Lanoxin)

SIDE EFFECTS

Edema	Drowsiness	URI
Nausea, constipation	Fatigue	Dizziness
Headache		

NURSING CONSIDERATIONS

- Management of hypertension and angina
- PO: take before meals, except sustained-release which is to be taken with food
- Do not open, chew, or crush sustained- or extended-release capsule
- Teach patient how to take radial pulse and keep records of pulse rate
- Avoid hazardous activities until stabilized on drug
- Do not use OTC products or alcohol unless directed by prescriber; limit caffeine
- Rx

• •

SIDE EFFECTS

Headache	Nausea	Dizziness
Hypotension	Atrial tachycardia	Mental disturbances
Fatigue	(in children)	Vomiting
Bradycardia		

NURSING CONSIDERATIONS

- Used in treatment of CHF, atrial fibrillation/flutter, or tachycardia
- Check pulse, if less than 60 beats per minute (adult) or 90 beats per minute (infant), hold the med and contact clinician
- PO: with or without food; may crush tablets and mix with food/fluids
- Do not open, chew, or crush capsule
- Contact clinician if loss of appetite, lower stomach pain, diarrhea, weakness, drowsiness, headache, blurred or yellow vision, rash, depression
- Eat a sodium-restricted and potassium-rich (bananas, orange juice) diet to keep potassium level normal
- Avoid OTC meds and herbal meds; many adverse interactions may occur
- Rx

BUMETANIDE
(byoo-<u>met</u>-a-nide)

• •

FUROSEMIDE
(fur-<u>oh</u>-se-mide)

(Lasix)

SIDE EFFECTS

Potassium depletion
Electrolyte
  imbalance
Hypovolemia

Ototoxicity
Hyperglycemia
Hypotension

Hives
Muscle weakness
Tinnitus

NURSING CONSIDERATIONS

- Treatment of edema, adult nocturia
- PO: diuresis onset 30–60 minutes, peak 1–2 hours, duration 3–6 hours
- IM: diuresis onset 40 minutes, peak 1–2 hours, duration 4–6 hours
- IV: diuresis onset 5 minutes, peak 15–30 minutes, duration 3–6 hours
- Weigh daily
- Do not take at bedtime to prevent nocturia
- Encourage potassium-containing foods
- May increase LDL, cholesterol, and triglycerides
- May increase HDL
- Monitor BUN, CBC, calcium, and uric acid
- Monitor for hearing loss
- Rx

• •

SIDE EFFECTS

Hypotension
Hypokalemia
Hyperglycemia
Nausea

Polyuria
Rash, pruritus
Muscle spasm

NURSING CONSIDERATIONS

- Used in treatment of pulmonary edema and edema in other conditions, hypertension
- PO: diuresis onset 60 minutes, peak 1–2 hours, duration 6–8 hours
- IV: diuresis onset 5 minutes, peak 30 minutes, duration 2 hours
- PO: take with food or milk to prevent GI upset, slightly lessened absorption, tablets may be crushed
- Take early in the day to prevent nocturia and sleeplessness
- Avoid changing positions (sitting/standing/lying) rapidly
- Use sunscreen or protective clothing to prevent photosensitivity
- NSAIDs may decrease effects
- Monitor blood sugar in diabetics
- Do not give IV faster than 4 mg/min; may cause ototoxicity
- Rx

CLOPIDOGREL
(klo-<u>pid</u>-oh-grel)

(Plavix)

• •

DIPYRIDAMOLE
(dye-peer-<u>id</u>-a-mole)

(Persantine)

SIDE EFFECTS

GI bleeding

Nausea, vomiting, diarrhea, GI
  discomfort

Depression

Bleeding, including
  life-threatening bleeding

Rash

NURSING CONSIDERATIONS

- Used to reduce risk of stroke, MI, peripheral artery disease in
  high-risk patients, ACS
- Monitor blood studies in long-term therapy
- Take with meals or just after to decrease gastric symptoms
- Report signs of unusual bruising, bleeding; it may take longer to
  stop bleeding
- Rx

• •

SIDE EFFECTS

Headache

Dizziness

Weakness, syncope

Nausea, vomiting

Postural hypotension

Rash

NURSING CONSIDERATIONS

- Prevention of transient ischemic attacks, MIs, with warfarin in
  heart valves, with ASA in bypass grafts
- PO: peak 2–2.5 hours; duration 6 hours
- PO: on an empty stomach, 1 hour before or 2 hours after meals
  with full glass of water
- Full therapeutic response may take several months
- IV: do not give more than 60 mg over 4 minutes
- Use caution with hazardous activities until stabilized on med
- Avoid changing positions (sitting/standing/lying) rapidly
- Intravenous aminophylline should be readily available to reverse
  effects of dipyridamole
- Rx

TICLOPIDINE HCL
(tye-<u>cloe</u>-pi-deen)

• •

HYDROCHLOROTHIAZIDE/ TRIAMTERENE
(hye-droe-klor-oh-<u>thye</u>-a-zide/
trye-<u>am</u>-ter-een)

(Dyazide, Maxzide)

SIDE EFFECTS

Rash
Diarrhea
Bleeding
Decrease in WBCs
Thrombocytopenia

Nausea
Dyspnea
GI distress
Purpura

NURSING CONSIDERATIONS

- Prevention of stroke in high-risk patients
- Monitor blood studies in long-term therapy
- Take with meals or just after to decrease gastric symptoms
- Monitor for signs of cholestasis (jaundice, dark urine, light-colored stools)
- May increase cholesterol and triglyceride levels
- Antacids may decrease effectiveness
- Rx

• •

SIDE EFFECTS

Nausea, vomiting, diarrhea
Anemia
Renal stones
Hyperkalemia

Hyperglycemia
Glycosuria
Muscle cramps

NURSING CONSIDERATIONS

- Used in treatment of edema and hypertension
- Diuresis onset 2 hours
- Take with meals or just after to decrease gastric symptoms
- Take early in the day to prevent nocturia and sleeplessness
- Diabetes mellitus may become manifest during thiazide treatment
- May increase BUN and serum creatinine
- Rx

SPIRONOLACTONE

(speer-in-oh-<u>lak</u>-tone)

(Aldactone)

• •

Cardiovascular Medications
Thiazides/Related Diuretics

CHLORTHALIDONE

(klor-<u>thal</u>-i-done)

(Thalitone, with atenolol Tenoretic)

SIDE EFFECTS

Hyperkalemia
Hyponatremia
Vomiting, diarrhea

Bleeding
Rash, pruritus
Gynecomastia

NURSING CONSIDERATIONS

- Used in treatment of edema and hypertension, primary hyperaldosteronism
- Diuresis onset 24–48 hours, peak 48–72 hours
- Take in the morning to avoid interference with sleep
- Take with meals or just after to decrease gastric symptoms
- Avoid food high in potassium: oranges, bananas, salt substitutes, dried apricots, dates
- Weigh daily to determine fluid loss; effect of drug may be decreased if used daily
- Contact clinician if cramps, lethargy, menstrual abnormalities, deepening voice, breast enlargement
- Avoid potassium supplements
- Monitor electrolytes
- Rx

• •

SIDE EFFECTS

Dizziness
Aplastic anemia
Orthostatic hypotension
Nausea, vomiting, anorexia

Urinary frequency
Fatigue, weakness
Electrolyte changes

NURSING CONSIDERATIONS

- Used in treatment of edema and hypertension
- Diuresis onset 2 hours, peak 6 hours, duration 24–72 hours
- Take with meals or just after to decrease gastric symptoms
- Blood sugar may increase in diabetics
- Take in the morning to avoid interference with sleep
- Weigh daily to determine fluid loss; effect of drug may be decreased if used daily
- May decrease PBI level
- Avoid changing positions (sitting/standing/lying) rapidly
- Rx

HYDROCHLOROTHIAZIDE
(hye-droe-klor-oh-<u>thye</u>-a-zide)

(Microzide)

· ·

INDAPAMIDE
(in-<u>dap</u>-a-mide)

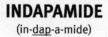

SIDE EFFECTS

Hypokalemia
Hyperglycemia
Nausea, vomiting, anorexia

Blurred vision
Fatigue, weakness
Confusion, esp. in elderly

NURSING CONSIDERATIONS

- Used in treatment of edema and hypertension
- Diuresis onset 2 hours, peak 4 hours, duration 6–12 hours
- Take with meals or just after to decrease gastric symptoms
- Blood sugar may increase in diabetics
- Take in morning to avoid interference with sleep
- Use sunscreen to prevent photosensitivity
- Monitor for signs of hypokalemia: postural hypotension, malaise, fatigue, tachycardia, leg cramps, weakness, dehydration
- Rx

• •

SIDE EFFECTS

Headache
Electrolyte changes
Orthostatic hypotension
Back pain
Gout
Muscle cramps

Cough
Rhinitis
Vision disturbances
Nausea
Rash, pruritus

NURSING CONSIDERATIONS

- Used in treatment of edema of CHF and hypertension
- Diuresis onset 1–2 hours, peak 2 hours, duration 36 hours
- Take with meals or just after to decrease gastric symptoms, slightly decreased absorption
- Avoid changing positions (sitting/standing/lying) rapidly
- Take in morning to avoid interference with sleep
- Monitor for signs of hypokalemia: postural hypotension, malaise, fatigue, tachycardia, leg cramps, weakness, dehydration
- Monitor electrolytes
- May cause hyperglycemia in diabetics
- Rx

METOLAZONE
(meh-<u>tole</u>-a-zone)

(Zaroxolyn—extended-release product)

· ·

Dermatologicals
Acne Agents, Oral

ISOTRETINOIN
(eye-sew-<u>tret</u>-i-noyn)

(Claravis)

SIDE EFFECTS

Dizziness, weakness, fatigue
Nausea, vomiting, anorexia
Rash

Hyperglycemia
Hypokalemia

NURSING CONSIDERATIONS

- Used in treatment of edema of CHF and hypertension, edema of renal diseases
- Diuresis onset 1 hour, peak 2 hours, duration 12–24 hours
- Take with meals or just after to decrease gastric symptoms, slightly decreased absorption
- Avoid changing positions (sitting/standing/lying) rapidly
- Take in morning to avoid interference with sleep
- Use sunscreen to prevent photosensitivity
- Monitor for signs of hypokalemia: postural hypotension, malaise, fatigue, tachycardia, leg cramps, weakness, dehydration
- May cause hyperglycemia in diabetics and latent diabetes
- Rx

• •

SIDE EFFECTS

Chilitis
Conjunctivitis
Dry skin
Dry mouth
Hair thinning

Cataracts
Aggression
Depression
Rash
Abnormal menses

NURSING CONSIDERATIONS

- Used to treat severe recalcitrant cystic acne that does not respond to conventional therapy, psoriasis, rosacea, basal cell carcinoma
- Women of child-bearing age must have a negative pregnancy test for each month of treatment
- Monitor for depression or suicidal thoughts
- Do not take vitamin A, may increase toxic effects
- Avoid St. John's wort
- June 2009, FDA pulled brand name Accutane
- October 2010, FDA issued warning to consumers not to buy isotretinoin over the Internet, due to lack of monitoring
- Rx

KETOCONAZOLE
(key-toe-<u>kon</u>-a-zole)

(Nizoral)

• •

NYSTATIN
(nye-<u>stat</u>-in)

(Mycostatin)

SIDE EFFECTS

Dizziness   Rash
Photophobia

NURSING CONSIDERATIONS

- Treatment of fungal infections
- C & S before first dose
- PO: take early A.M. with food
- Also available as a topical cream or shampoo
- Cannot take within 2 hours of alkaline substances, requires acid media to dissolve, follow with glass of water
- Take at the same time each day
- To prevent photophobia in bright sunlight, wear sunglasses
- May require several weeks or months of therapy
- Avoid alcohol
- Do not allow shampoo to get in eyes
- Rx

• •

SIDE EFFECTS

GI distress, hypersensitivity
Irritation (with topical use)

NURSING CONSIDERATIONS

- Treatment of *Candida* infections
- Discontinue if redness, swelling, irritation occurs
- Encourage good oral, vaginal, skin hygiene
- Do not mix oral suspension with food
- Rx

FLUOCINONIDE
(floo-oh-<u>sin</u>-oh-nide)

(Lidex)

• •

TRIAMCINOLONE ACETONIDE
(try-am-<u>sin</u>-oh-lone)

(Kenalog)

SIDE EFFECTS

Acne	Striae
Atrophy	Burning
Epidermal thinning	Allergic dermatitis
Purpura	

NURSING CONSIDERATIONS

- Topical glucocorticoid used to treat severe dermatoses not responding to less potent meds: psoriasis, eczema, contact dermatitis, pruritus
- Apply only to affected areas; do not get in eyes
- Leave site uncovered or lightly covered
- Occlusive dressing is not recommended, systemic absorption may occur
- Do not use on weeping, denuded, or infected areas
- Avoid sunlight on affected area
- Rx

• •

SIDE EFFECTS

Acne	Striae
Atrophy	Allergic contact dermatitis
Epidermal thinning	Hypopigmentation
Purpura	

NURSING CONSIDERATIONS

- Topical glucocorticoid used to treat severe dermatoses not responding to less potent meds: psoriasis, eczema, contact dermatitis, pruritus
- Apply only to affected areas; do not get in eyes
- Leave site uncovered or lightly covered
- Occlusive dressing is not recommended, systemic absorption may occur
- Do not use on weeping, denuded, or infected areas
- Avoid sunlight on affected area
- Rx

EXENATIDE
(ex-<u>en</u>-a-tide)

(Byetta, Bydureon)

. . . .

Diabetic Medications
Hypoglycemic Agents, Oral

ACARBOSE
(ay-<u>car</u>-bose)

(Precose)

SIDE EFFECTS

Nausea

Vomiting

Diarrhea

Constipation

Gastroparesis

Injection site reactions

Hypoglycemia

Pancreatitis

Headache

Dizziness

Decreased appetite/weight loss

NURSING CONSIDERATIONS

- Used for the treatment of type 2 diabetes mellitus
- SubQ: give extended-release product once weekly without regard to food; give immediate-release product twice daily 30 minutes before a meal
- Extended-release version requires reconstitution just before administration
- Both products are refrigerated before use
- Do not use in patients with severe renal impairment or history of pancreatitis
- Routinely monitor blood glucose
- Rx

• •

SIDE EFFECTS

Abdominal pain

Diarrhea

Flatulence

Rash

NURSING CONSIDERATIONS

- Management of diabetes by non-insulin-dependent diabetics
- Used alone or in combination with a sulfonylurea or insulin
- PO: take with first bite of each meal, med blood level peaks in 1 hour
- Recognize signs of hypoglycemia: weakness, hunger, dizziness, tremors, anxiety, tachycardia, hunger, sweating
- Treat hypoglycemia with dextrose, or if severe, IV glucose or glucagon
- Measure short-term effectiveness with blood sugar 1 hour after meals
- Measure long-term effectiveness with glycosylated Hgb every 3 months for the first year
- Wear medical information tag
- Rx

GLIMEPIRIDE
(glye-<u>meh</u>-pi-ride)

(Amaryl)

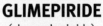

Diabetic Medications
Hypoglycemic Agents, Oral

GLIPIZIDE
(<u>glip</u>-i-zide)

(Glucotrol)

SIDE EFFECTS

Headache

Dyspnea

Weakness, dizziness

Fall in blood pressure

Drowsiness

Shock

NURSING CONSIDERATIONS

- Management of stable type 2 diabetes mellitus
- Do not drink alcohol since it may produce a disulfiram reaction: nausea, headache, cramps, flushing, hypoglycemia
- Assess for symptoms of cholestatic jaundice: dark urine, pruritus, yellow sclera (rare)
- Take at breakfast or first main meal; onset 1–1.5 hours, peak 1–3 hours, duration 10–24 hours
- Have a quick source of sugar or a glucagon emergency kit available
- Use sunscreen or protective clothing to prevent photosensitivity
- Do not crush, chew, or break extended-release tablet; its coating may appear in stool
- Cross-allergy possible if allergic to sulfonamide
- Monitor blood sugars
- Wear medical information tag
- Rx

• •

SIDE EFFECTS

Headache

Dizziness

Weakness

Drowsiness

NURSING CONSIDERATIONS

- Management of adults with type 2 diabetes mellitus
- Do not drink alcohol since it can produce a disulfiram reaction: nausea, headache, cramps, flushing, hypoglycemia
- Assess for symptoms of cholestatic jaundice: dark urine, pruritus, yellow sclera (rare)
- Take at breakfast; onset 1–1.5 hours, peak 1–3 hours, duration 10–24 hours
- Immediate-release: take 30 minutes before meals, since absorption is delayed by food
- Have a quick source of sugar or a glucagon emergency kit available
- Use sunscreen or protective clothing to prevent photosensitivity
- Extended-release tablet coating may appear in stool
- May cause hemolytic anemia when used with sulfonylurea agents
- Monitor blood sugar
- Wear medical information tag
- Rx

GLYBURIDE
(<u>glye</u>-byoo-ride)

(DiaBeta)

. . . .

METFORMIN HCL
(met-<u>for</u>-min)

(Glucophage)

SIDE EFFECTS

Headache

Weakness, dizziness

GI disturbances

Allergic skin reactions

NURSING CONSIDERATIONS

- Management of adult type 2 diabetes mellitus
- Assess for symptoms of cholestatic jaundice: dark urine, pruritus, yellow sclera (rare)
- Take at breakfast; onset 2–4 hours, peak 4 hours, duration 24 hours
- Have a quick source of sugar or a glucagon emergency kit available
- Use sunscreen or protective clothing to prevent photosensitivity
- May cause hemolytic anemia in some patients
- Monitor blood sugar
- Wear medical information tag
- Rx

• •

SIDE EFFECTS

Headache

Weakness, dizziness, drowsiness

Agitation

Nausea, vomiting, diarrhea

Lactic acidosis

Flatulence

NURSING CONSIDERATIONS

- Management of adult type 2 diabetes mellitus
- PO: twice a day with meals to decrease GI upset and provide best absorption; may also be taken as one dose
- Can crush tablets and mix with juice or soft foods for ease of swallowing
- Do not crush, chew, or break extended-release tablet; its coating may appear in stool
- Be aware of signs of lactic acidosis: hyperventilation, fatigue, malaise, chills, myalgia, sleepiness
- Have a quick source of sugar or a glucagon emergency kit available
- Monitor blood sugar
- Wear medical information tag
- Rx

PIOGLITAZONE HCL
(pye-oh-gli-ta-zone)

(Actos)

. . . .

SITAGLIPTIN
(sye-ta-glip-tin)

(Januvia)

SIDE EFFECTS

Cold symptoms

Respiratory infection

Headache

Muscle pain

Sinusitis

Tooth disorder

NURSING CONSIDERATIONS

- Treatment of type 2 diabetes
- Take around the same time each day, once daily, with or without food
- Full therapeutic effects may require 2 or more weeks
- Used in conjunction with diet and exercise regimen
- May exacerbate CHF; monitor for edema and lung sounds
- Monitor liver enzymes
- Patient should have regular eye exams for macular edema
- May increase risk of bone fractures
- August 2011, FDA issued alert: use of drug for more than 1 year is associated with increased risk of bladder cancer
- Rx

• •

SIDE EFFECTS

Pancreatitis

Headache

Kidney problems, sometimes
  requiring dialysis

Rhinitis

Sore throat

Upper respiratory infection

NURSING CONSIDERATIONS

- Used to lower blood pressure levels in adults with type 2 diabetes
- Used in conjunction with diet and exercise regimen
- Teach patient how to monitor blood sugar
- Medication should be taken immediately before a meal
- Contact prescriber immediately if symptoms of pancreatitis (persistent, severe abdominal pain with or without vomiting)
- Rx

INSULIN ASPART
(NovoLog)

• •

INSULIN GLARGINE
(Lantus, Lantus Solostar)

SIDE EFFECTS

Hypoglycemia	Headache
Lipodystrophy	Weight gain
Hypokalemia	Edema
Allergic reactions	

NURSING CONSIDERATIONS

- Management of diabetes in adults; the only insulin analog approved for use in external pump systems for continuous subQ insulin infusion
- Onset 15 minutes, peak 1–3 hours, duration 3–5 hours
- May be administered IV in emergency situations under medical supervision with close blood-sugar monitoring
- Immediately follow injection with meal within 5–10 minutes
- Rx

· ·

SIDE EFFECTS

Hypoglycemia	Pruritus
Lipodystrophy	Rash
Allergic reactions	

NURSING CONSIDERATIONS

- Management of diabetes in type 1 diabetics or adults with type 2 requiring a long-acting insulin to control hyperglycemia
- No pronounced peak, duration 24 hours
- Must inject at same time each day
- Not the drug of choice for diabetic ketoacidosis (use a short-acting insulin)
- Higher incidence of injection site pain compared with NPH insulin
- Monitor blood sugar
- Do not administer IV or via insulin pump
- Do not mix with any other insulin
- Rx

INSULIN-ISOPHANE SUSPENSION (NPH)
(Humulin N, Novolin N)

• •

INSULIN LISPRO
(Humalog)

SIDE EFFECTS

Hypoglycemia   Allergic reactions
Lipodystrophy

NURSING CONSIDERATIONS

- Management of diabetes
- Comes in 100 units per milliliter vial, as well as in combination with regular insulin in a 50/50 proportion and 75/25 proportion
- subQ: onset 1–1.5 hours, peak 4–12 hours, duration 18–24 hours
- Read administration instructions carefully
- Do not give IV
- Monitor blood sugar
- OTC, Rx

. . . .

SIDE EFFECTS

Hypoglycemia   Allergic reactions
Lipodystrophy

NURSING CONSIDERATIONS

- Management of type 1 diabetes and in combination with sulfonylureas for type 2 diabetes
- Take within 15 minutes of eating and immediately after mixing, with combined therapy
- May be used in children in combination with sulfonylureas
- Onset rapid, peak 30–90 minutes, duration 6–8 hours
- May be used in an external insulin pump
- Monitor blood sugar
- May be administered IV in emergency situations under medical supervision with close blood-sugar monitoring
- If administered using insulin pen, read instructions carefully
- Do not mix with other insulins
- Available in combination with other insulin
- Rx

INSULIN, REGULAR
(Humulin R)

• •

Diabetic Medications
Reversal of Hypoglycemia

GLUCAGON
(gloo-ka-gon)
(GlucaGen)

SIDE EFFECTS

Hypoglycemia   Allergic reaction
Lipodystrophy   Hypokalemia

NURSING CONSIDERATIONS

- Management of diabetic coma, diabetic acidosis, or other emergency conditions; esp. suitable for labile diabetes
- Comes in 100 units/milliliter vial
- Only insulin that can be given IV in non-emergency situations
- subQ: onset 30–60 minutes, peak 2–3 hours, duration 3–6 hours
- IV: onset 10–30 minutes, peak 10–30 minutes, duration 30–60 minutes
- Read insulin pen instructions carefully
- May be mixed with NPH only in same syringe; draw Novolin R first
- Do not use in insulin pumps
- Monitor blood sugar
- Do not rub site after subQ injection
- OTC, Rx

• •

SIDE EFFECTS

Nausea, vomiting

NURSING CONSIDERATIONS

- Acute management of severe hypoglycemia; facilitation of GI x-rays
- IM for hypoglycemia: onset within 10 minutes, peak 30 minutes, duration 60–90 minutes
- IV for hypoglycemia: onset within 10 minutes, peak 5 minutes, duration 60–90 minutes
- subQ for hypoglycemia: onset within 10 minutes, peak 30–45 minutes, duration 60–90 minutes
- IV for GI x-rays: onset within 45 seconds, duration dosedependent of 9–25 minutes
- IM for GI x-rays: onset within 8–10 minutes, duration dosedependent of 9–32 minutes
- Monitor blood sugar until patient is asymptomatic
- Use reconstituted mixture within 15 minutes of mix
- OTC, Rx

ALUMINUM HYDROXIDE GEL
(Amphojel)

• •

CALCIUM CARBONATE
(Tums)

SIDE EFFECTS

Constipation that may lead to impaction

Phosphate depletion

NURSING CONSIDERATIONS

- Antacid; used in renal failure to control hyperphosphatemia because drug contains aluminum, which binds with phosphate in the GI tract
- PO: shake suspension well, follow with small amount of milk or water to facilitate passage; duration 20–180 minutes
- Contact clinician if signs of GI bleeding: tarry stools, coffee-grounds vomitus
- Monitor long-term, high-dose use if on restricted sodium intake, due to high sodium content
- If prolonged use, monitor for phosphate depletion: anorexia, malaise, and muscle weakness; can also lead to resorption of calcium and bone demineralization in uremia patients
- Do not take longer than 2 weeks
- Aluminum antacid compounds interfere with tetracycline absorption
- Use may interfere with some imaging techniques
- Rx

• •

SIDE EFFECTS

Nausea
Anorexia
Constipation

Dry mouth
Possible allergic reaction

NURSING CONSIDERATIONS

- Used as antacid and calcium supplement
- May decrease effect of some antibiotics and other drugs due to impaired absorption, so separate administration times by 2 hours
- Do not use if ventricular fibrillation or hypercalcemia
- Use caution if taking cardiac glycoside or has sarcoidosis or renal or cardiac disease
- Signs of hypercalcemia: nausea, vomiting, headache, confusion, anorexia
- OTC

MAGALDRATE
(<u>mag</u>-al-drate)
(Riopan)

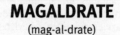

Gastrointestinal Medications
Anticholinergics

DICYCLOMINE HCL
(dye-<u>sye</u>-kloh-meen)
(Bentyl)

SIDE EFFECTS

Mild constipation

Increased urine pH levels

Diarrhea

Hypophosphatemia

NURSING CONSIDERATIONS

- Symptomatic relief of GERD, indigestion, and GI distress
- Shake suspension well and follow with small amount of water to facilitate passage
- Onset 20 minutes, duration 20–180 minutes
- May decrease effect of antibiotics and other drugs, such as digoxin, phenothiazines, quinidine, salicylates due to impaired absorption, so separate administration times by 1–2 hours
- Because low sodium content, used in patients on sodium restriction
- If given with enteric-coated drugs, might have premature release in stomach; separate administration times by at least 1 hour
- Contact clinician if signs of GI bleeding: tarry stools or coffeegrounds vomitus
- Rx

· ·

SIDE EFFECTS

Drowsiness

Blurred vision

Dyspnea

Dry mouth

Rash

Urinary hesitancy

Tachycardia

Headache

NURSING CONSIDERATIONS

- Used for treatment of irritable bowel syndrome
- Take 30 minutes before meals and at bedtime
- Use caution with potentially hazardous activities
- Report diarrhea—may be incomplete intestinal obstruction
- Rx

HYOSCYAMINE
(hye-oh-<u>sye</u>-a-meen)

(Anaspaz, Gastrosed)

• •

Gastrointestinal Medications
Antidiarrheals

LOPERAMIDE HCL
(loe-<u>per</u>-a-mide)

(Imodium)

SIDE EFFECTS

Confusion, stimulation in
  elderly
Dry mouth, constipation
Urinary retention, hesitancy
Palpitations

Blurred vision
Tachycardia
Rash
Headache
Drowsiness

NURSING CONSIDERATIONS

- Treatment of peptic ulcer, other GI disorders, other spastic disorders, urinary incontinence
- PO: onset 20–30 minutes, duration 4–6 hours
- IM, IV, subQ: onset 2–3 minutes, duration 4–6 hours
- Avoid activities requiring alertness until stabilized on med
- Avoid alcohol, CNS depressants
- Use sunglasses to prevent photophobia
- Take 30–60 minutes before meals
- Avoid antacids within 1 hour
- Rx

• •

SIDE EFFECTS

Nausea, vomiting
Abdominal pain/distention
Dizziness

Drowsiness
Dry mouth

NURSING CONSIDERATIONS

- Used for control of diarrhea, including diarrhea in travelers
- Take with a full glass of water
- Encourage 6–8 glasses of fluid per day
- Use caution with potentially hazardous activities
- If abdominal distention in acute ulcerative colitis, stop med
- Avoid use with alcohol, CNS depressants
- Follow clear liquid or bland diet until diarrhea subsides
- Do not use OTC if fever over 101°F (38°C) or if bloody diarrhea
- OTC, Rx

MECLIZINE
(<u>mek</u>-li-zeen)

(Antivert, Bonine)

METOCLOPRAMIDE HCL
(met-oh-<u>kloe</u>-pra-mide)

(Reglan)

SIDE EFFECTS

Drowsiness
Dizziness

NURSING CONSIDERATIONS

- Management of vertigo, motion sickness
- Duration 8–14 hours
- Take 1 hour before traveling
- Avoid activities requiring alertness
- Avoid alcohol, CNS depressants
- OTC, Rx

• •

SIDE EFFECTS

Drowsiness	Sleeplessness
Restlessness	Dry mouth
Lassitude	Anxiety
Headache	

NURSING CONSIDERATIONS

- Prevention of nausea, vomiting induced by chemotherapy, radiation, delayed gastric emptying, GERD
- Used with tube feeding to decrease residual and risk of aspiration
- PO: take 30–60 minutes before meals or procedures
- IV: inject slowly over 1–2 minutes; infuse over 15 minutes
- Use caution with potentially hazardous activities
- Avoid alcohol, CNS depressants
- May cause tardive dyskinesia
- May cause depression
- Rx

PROCHLORPERAZINE
(proe-klor-<u>pair</u>-a-zeen)

(Compro)

• •

PROMETHAZINE
(pro-<u>meth</u>-a-zeen)

(Phenergan)

SIDE EFFECTS

Orthostatic hypotension
Blurred vision
Dry eyes, dry mouth

Constipation
Drowsiness
Photosensitivity

NURSING CONSIDERATIONS

- Management of nausea, vomiting, psychotic disorders
- Monitor for development of neuroleptic malignant syndrome (fever, respiratory distress, tachycardia, convulsions, sweating, hypertension or hypotension, pallor, tiredness, severe muscle stiffness, loss of bladder control); notify clinician immediately
- PO: take with food
- Do not crush or break sustained-release capsules
- IM: inject slowly, deeply into gluteal UOQ; keep patient lying down for 30 minutes
- Use caution with potentially hazardous activities
- Avoid changing positions (lying/sitting/standing) rapidly
- Wear sunscreen and protective clothing to prevent photosensitivity reactions
- Check CBC and liver functions with prolonged use
- Risk of increase mortality in elderly patients with dementia; related psychosis
- May develop tardive dyskinesia
- Rx

• •

SIDE EFFECTS

Drowsiness
Dizziness
Constipation

Urinary retention
Dry mouth
Hyperglycemia

NURSING CONSIDERATIONS

- Management of motion sickness, rhinitis, allergy symptoms, sedation, nausea, pre- and postoperative sedation
- PO: onset 20 minutes, duration 4–6 hours
- Take 30–60 minutes before traveling
- Avoid activities requiring alertness
- Avoid alcohol, CNS depressants
- May cause severe chemical irritation and damage to tissue
- May lower seizure threshold
- May cause false results in pregnancy testing
- Rx

SIMETHICONE
(si-<u>meth</u>-i-kone)

. . . .

Gastrointestinal Medications
Antisecretory

ESOMEPRAZOLE MAGNESIUM
(e-sew-<u>mep</u>-ruh-zole)

(Nexium)

SIDE EFFECTS
Belching
Rectal flatus

NURSING CONSIDERATIONS
- Helps disperse gas pockets in GI system, does not decrease gas production
- Take after meals, at bedtime
- Shake suspension well before pouring
- Tablets must be chewed
- OTC, Rx

• •

SIDE EFFECTS

Headache	Flatulence
Diarrhea	Dry mouth
Nausea	

NURSING CONSIDERATIONS
- Short-term treatment of erosive esophagitis
- Used to treat GERD
- Take at least 60 minutes before meals
- Swallow capsules whole, do not chew
- May be taken in conjunction with antacids
- Rx

OMEPRAZOLE

(oh-<u>meh</u>-pruh-zole)

(Prilosec)

· ·

Gastrointestinal Medications
Antiulcer Medications

CIMETIDINE

(sye-<u>met</u>-ih-deen)

(Tagamet)

SIDE EFFECTS

Headache   Flatulence
Nausea, vomiting, diarrhea

NURSING CONSIDERATIONS

- Treatment of active duodenal ulcers
- Treatment of GERD in patients over age 2 years
- Take 30 minutes before eating
- May be taken at the same time as antacids
- OTC, Rx

• •

SIDE EFFECTS

Diarrhea   Headache
Confusion (esp. in elderly with   Dysrhythmias
  large doses)

NURSING CONSIDERATIONS

- Treatment of ulcers; may be used for prevention of
  aspiration pneumonia, stress ulcers, idiopathic urticaria,
  hyperparathyroidism
- Reduces gastric acid secretions by 50%–80%
- May be taken without regard to meals
- Avoid antacids 1 hour before or after dose
- Do not use OTC for more than 2 weeks unless medically
  supervised; avoid use under age 12
- Monitor liver enzymes and blood counts
- OTC, Rx

FAMOTIDINE
(fa-<u>moe</u>-ti-deen)

(Pepcid)

• •

LANSOPRAZOLE
(lan-<u>soe</u>-pra-zole)

(Prevacid)

SIDE EFFECTS

Headache
Blood dyscrasias
Hepatitis

Dizziness
Constipation

NURSING CONSIDERATIONS

- Treatment of duodenal and gastric ulcers, GERD, heartburn
- PO: onset 30–60 minutes, peak 1–3 hours, duration 6–12 hours
- IV: onset immediate, peak 30–60 minutes, duration 8–15 hours
- Signs of blood dyscrasia: bleeding, bruising, fatigue, malaise, poor healing, jaundice
- OTC, Rx

. . . .

SIDE EFFECTS

Dizziness
Diarrhea

Abdominal pain

NURSING CONSIDERATIONS

- Used for treatment of GERD and ulcers, erosive esophagitis
- PO: take no more than 30 minutes before meals; capsules may be opened and sprinkled on food (applesauce, pudding, cottage cheese, yogurt) and swallowed immediately
- Can use with antacids
- Do not crush or chew capsule contents
- To give with NG tube in place, open the capsule and mix with orange, apple or tomato juice, instill through NG tube and flush with additional juice to clear tube
- Report severe diarrhea
- Rx

MISOPROSTOL

(mye-soe-<u>prost</u>-ole)

(Cytotec)

• •

RABEPRAZOLE

(rah-<u>bep</u>-rah-zole)

(AcipHex)

SIDE EFFECTS

Abdominal pain   Nausea
Diarrhea   Headache
Miscarriage

NURSING CONSIDERATIONS

- Prevention of gastric ulcers during NSAID therapy
- Take with meals and at bedtime
- Avoid taking magnesium antacids within 2 hours
- Notify clinician if diarrhea lasts more than 1 week
- Notify clinician if black, tarry stools or severe abdominal pain
- Rx

• •

SIDE EFFECTS

Headache   Constipation, flatulence
Dizziness   Rash
Nausea, vomiting, diarrhea   Back pain

NURSING CONSIDERATIONS

- Used for treatment of GERD and duodenal ulcers
- Take on an empty stomach before eating
- Swallow tablets whole; do not crush, chew, or split tablets
- Avoid alcohol, NSAIDs, and ASA; may increase gastric upset
- Rx

RANITIDINE
(ra-<u>nit</u>-i-deen)

(Zantac)

• •

SUCRALFATE
(soo-<u>kral</u>-fate)

(Carafate)

SIDE EFFECTS

Dizziness (esp. in elderly)   Headache
Drowsiness

NURSING CONSIDERATIONS

- Used to inhibit gastric acid secretion, ulcers (GI)
- Take with or immediately following meals
- Do not take antacids within 1 hour before or after
- Do not smoke; it interferes with healing and drug's effectiveness
- Avoid alcohol, ASA, and caffeine, which increase stomach acid
- False positive tests for urine protein may occur
- OTC, Rx

• •

SIDE EFFECTS

Constipation
Hypersensitivity

NURSING CONSIDERATIONS

- Short-term treatment (less than 8 weeks) of duodenal ulcers
- PO: 1 hour before meals or 2 hours after meals and at bedtime
  with full glass of water
- Do not chew tablets
- Do not use antacids within 30 minutes of med
- Encourage 8–10 glasses of fluid per day
- Avoid smoking
- Rx

SULFASALAZINE
(sul-fah-<u>sal</u>-a-zeen)

(Azulfidine)

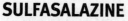

PHENTERMINE
(<u>fen</u>-ter-meen)

(Ionamin)

SIDE EFFECTS

Headache
Anorexia
Nausea, vomiting, diarrhea
Rashes

Fever
Oligospermia
Hepatotoxicity

NURSING CONSIDERATIONS

- Used for treatment of inflammatory bowel diseases and arthritis
- PO: take with food to decrease GI upset
- Encourage fluids to decrease crystallization in kidneys
- May permanently stain contact lens yellow
- May cause orange-yellow urine and skin, which is not significant
- Wear sunscreen and protective clothing to prevent photosensitivity reactions
- Monitor liver enzymes
- Rx

• •

SIDE EFFECTS

CNS stimulation
Hypertension
Changes in libido

Palpitations
Drowsiness

NURSING CONSIDERATIONS

- Short-term treatment of obesity
- PO, hydrochloride form: duration 4 hours
- PO, resin complex form: duration 12–14 hours
- Take 30 minutes before meals or as a single dose before breakfast or 10–14 hours before bedtime
- Avoid activities requiring alertness until response is known
- Avoid alcohol, CNS depressants
- Contact clinician if chest pain, decreased exercise tolerance, fainting, or lower extremity swelling
- Controlled Substance Schedule IV

LACTULOSE SYRUP
(<u>lak</u>-tyoo-lose)

(Enulose)

· ·

PANCRELIPASE
(pan-kre-<u>li</u>-pase)

(Pancrease, Viokase)

SIDE EFFECTS

Nausea, vomiting
Abdominal cramps

NURSING CONSIDERATIONS

- Used for chronic constipation; prevention and treatment of portal-systemic encephalotic including hepatic precoma and coma
- PO: take with water or fruit juice to counteract sweet taste
- Use with caution in diabetics
- Monitor blood sugar
- Rx

• •

SIDE EFFECTS

Abdominal pain
 (high doses only)
Nausea, diarrhea
Stomach cramps

Flatulence
Abnormal feces
Fatigue

NURSING CONSIDERATIONS

- Used to replace or supplement naturally occurring enzymes; contains lipase, amylase, and protease lost due to cystic fibrosis Take with 8 ounces of water and food, swallow right away, sit up when taking
- Do not crush or break enteric-coated capsules
- Do not use if sensitive or allergy to pork
- Stools will be foul-smelling and frothy
- Rx

Genitourinary Medications
Alpha-Adrenoceptor Antagonist

TAMSULOSIN HCL
(tam-sull-<u>oh</u>-sin)

(Flomax)

• •

Genitourinary Medications
Anticholinergics

OXYBUTYNIN CHLORIDE
(ox-i-<u>byoo</u>-ti-nin)

(Ditropan)

SIDE EFFECTS

Sleepiness, difficulty falling or
  staying asleep
Weakness
Back pain
Nausea, vomiting, diarrhea
UTI
Cold symptoms, including pain
  or pressure in the face

Blurred vision
Abnormal ejaculation
Dizziness
Headache
Increased cough
Chest pain
Priapism

NURSING CONSIDERATIONS

- Treatment of benign prostatic hyperplasia
- Take the same time daily, once a day, 30 minutes after a meal
- Avoid changing positions (lying, sitting, standing) rapidly
- Use caution in potentially hazardous activities
- May have cross-allergy with sulfa drugs
- This medication should be stopped prior to cataract surgery;
  may cause IFIS
- Rx

• •

SIDE EFFECTS

Anxiety, restlessness
Dizziness
Convulsions
Palpitations, tachycardia
Drowsiness, blurred vision

Nausea, vomiting
Anorexia
Dry mouth
Mydriasis
Constipation

NURSING CONSIDERATIONS

- Antispasmodic treatment of neurogenic bladder
- Take on an empty stomach
- Avoid alcohol, CNS depressants
- Avoid activities requiring alertness until med response is known
- Decreased ability to perspire; avoid strenuous activity in warm
  weather
- Wear sunglasses in bright sunlight to prevent photophobia
- Rx

TOLTERODINE TARTRATE
(toal-<u>tair</u>-oh-deen)

(Detrol, Detrol LA)

. . . .

SILDENAFIL CITRATE
(sil-<u>den</u>-a-fill)

(Viagra)

SIDE EFFECTS

Dry mouth
Dizziness
Constipation

Dyspepsia
Somnolence
Blurred vision

NURSING CONSIDERATIONS

- Used to treat patients with overactive bladder
- Effective with frequency, urgency, or incontinence symptoms
- Patients should avoid alcohol during treatment with tolterodine
- Missed doses should be skipped, return to normal schedule
- Rx

• •

SIDE EFFECTS

Headache, flushing
Dizziness
Upset stomach
Nasal congestion
UTI

Abnormal vision
Rash
Tinnitus, hearing loss
Visual disturbances

NURSING CONSIDERATIONS

- Treatment of erectile dysfunction
- Take approximately 1 hour before sexual activity
- Do not use more than once a day
- Tablets may be split
- High-fat meal will reduce absorption; better absorption on empty stomach
- Never use with nitrates; could have fatal fall in blood pressure
- Notify clinician if erection lasts longer than 4 hours
- Stop medication if hearing or visual disturbances occur
- Rx

TADALAFIL
(teh-<u>dal</u>-uh-fil)

(Cialis)

• •

VARDENAFIL
(var-<u>den</u>-uh-fil)

(Levitra)

SIDE EFFECTS

Headache
Dyspepsia
Back pain

Tinnitus, hearing loss
Myalgia
Nasal congestion

NURSING CONSIDERATIONS

- Used to treat erectile dysfunction
- Patients with severe hepatic impairment should not take tadalafil
- Contraindicated in patients taking nitrates or alpha-adrenergic blockers
- Tadalafil does not protect against sexually transmitted diseases
- Alert physician if erection lasts more than 4 hours
- Stop medication if hearing or visual disturbances occur
- Alcohol intake may increase orthostatic symptoms
- Rx

• •

SIDE EFFECTS

Headache
Nasal congestion
Flushing

Dyspepsia
Tinnitus, hearing loss

NURSING CONSIDERATIONS

- Used to treat erectile dysfunction
- Contraindicated in patients taking organic nitrates
- Contact physician if erection lasts over 4 hours
- Plasma levels peak in 30 minutes to 2 hours
- Stop medication if hearing or visual disturbances occur
- Alpha blocker used with this medication may cause syncope
- Rx

FINASTERIDE
(fin-<u>as</u>-teh-ride)

(Proscar, Propecia)

• •

PHENAZOPYRIDINE HCL
(fen-az-oh-<u>peer</u>-i-deen)

(Pyridium)

SIDE EFFECTS

Decreased libido
Decreased volume of ejaculate
Testicular pain
Impotence

Breast tenderness and
  enlargement
Angioedema

NURSING CONSIDERATIONS

- Treatment of BPH by Proscar, male hair loss by Propecia
- May be taken without regard to food
- Pregnant women should avoid contact with crushed drug or patient's semen; may adversely affect developing male fetus
- Full therapeutic effect: Propecia may require 3 months, Proscar may require 6–12 months
- Not for use in women and children
- Rx

• •

SIDE EFFECTS

GI upset
Kidney and liver toxicity

Rash
Headache

NURSING CONSIDERATIONS

- Treatment of urinary tract irritation, often paired with urinary anti-infective
- Do not crush tablets; can take with food or milk to decrease GI upset
- Inform patient that urine will be bright orange/red
- Monitor for signs of hepatoxicity: dark urine, clay-colored stools, jaundice, itching, abdominal pain, fever, diarrhea
- May interfere with urine glucose tests
- OTC, Rx

NITROFURANTOIN

(nye-troe-<u>fyoor</u>-an-toyn)

(Furadantin, Macrobid, Macrodantin)

• •

Hormones/Synthetic Substitutes/Modifiers
Bone Resorption Inhibitors

ALENDRONATE

(al-en-<u>drone</u>-ate)

(Fosamax)

SIDE EFFECTS

Dizziness
Nausea, vomiting, diarrhea
Abdominal pain

Tooth staining
Hypersensitivity

NURSING CONSIDERATIONS

- Treatment of UTIs
- Take with food or milk
- Avoid alcohol
- Two daily doses if urine output is high or patient has diabetes
- Drug may turn urine rust-yellow to brown
- May cause false positive glucose in urine
- May increase AST and ALT
- Rx

• •

SIDE EFFECTS

Esophageal ulceration
GI distress

Musculoskeletal pain

NURSING CONSIDERATIONS

- Prevention and treatment of osteoporosis in women; treatment of osteoporosis in men; treatment of Paget disease
- Onset: 1 month, peak 3–6 months, duration 3 weeks to 7 months
- Take in A.M. before food or other meds with full glass of water; remain upright for 30 minutes
- If dose missed, skip dose; do not double dose or take later in the day
- Take with calcium and vitamin D if instructed by clinician
- May cause atypical subtrochanteric femur fractures
- Rx

RISEDRONATE

(riss-<u>ed</u>-roe-nate)

(Actonel)

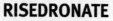

Hormones/Synthetic Substitutes/Modifiers
Parathyroid Agents (Calcium Regulators)

ETIDRONATE

(eh-tih-<u>droe</u>-nate)

(Didronel)

SIDE EFFECTS

Weakness

Diarrhea, abdominal pain

Bone pain

Back pain

Joint pain

Dyspepsia

Hypersensitivity

Eye inflammation

NURSING CONSIDERATIONS

- Prevention and treatment of osteoporosis in women; treatment of osteoporosis in men; treatment of Paget disease
- Onset: within days, peak 30 days, duration up to 16 months
- Take in A.M. before food or other meds with full glass of water; remain upright for 30 minutes
- Take with calcium and vitamin D if instructed by clinician
- May cause atypical subtrochanteric femur fractures
- Rx

- -

SIDE EFFECTS

Nausea, diarrhea

Bone pain and tenderness

Myalgia

Hypersensitivity

Headache

Arthralgia

NURSING CONSIDERATIONS

- Treatment of Paget disease, used with total hip replacement and spinal cord injury, hyperkalemia of cancer
- PO: onset 1 month, duration 1 year
- IV: onset 24 hours, peak 3 days, duration 11 days
- Take on empty stomach with calcium and vitamin D, but not within 2 hours of med
- Contact clinician if sudden onset of unexpected pain, restricted mobility, heat over bone
- May cause atypical subtrochanteric femur fractures
- Rx

THYROID, DESICCATED
(<u>thigh</u>-roid)

(Armour Thyroid)

• •

LEVOTHYROXINE (T4)
(lee-voe-thye-<u>rox</u>-een)

(Synthroid, Levothroid)

SIDE EFFECTS

Weight loss
Palpitations
Diarrhea

Tachycardia
Sweating

NURSING CONSIDERATIONS

- Used to treat adult hypothyroidism
- Side effects are rare and generally associated with overdosing
- Dosed at 15–30 mg initially and titrated up every 2–3 weeks until optimum results are present
- Thyroid levels should be checked every 6 months after patient is stabilized
- Patient should avoid OTC preparations and food with iodine
- Rx

• •

SIDE EFFECTS

Weight loss
Arrhythmias, tachycardia
Insomnia, irritability

Nervousness
Heat intolerance
Menstrual irregularities

NURSING CONSIDERATIONS

- Management of hypothyroidism, myxedema coma, thyroid hormone replacement
- PO: peak 1–3 weeks, duration 1–3 weeks
- IV: onset 6–8 hours, peak 24 hours
- PO: take at same time daily to maintain blood level; take on empty stomach
- Do not switch brands unless directed
- Avoid OTC meds with iodine and iodized salt, soybeans, tofu, turnips, walnuts, some seafood, some bread
- Drug is not a cure, but controls symptoms and treatment is lifelong
- Rx

ALPRAZOLAM
(al-<u>pray</u>-zoe-lam)

(Xanax)

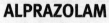

BUSPIRONE
(byoo-<u>spye</u>-rone)

(BuSpar)

SIDE EFFECTS

Dizziness, drowsiness
Orthostatic hypotension

Blurred vision

NURSING CONSIDERATIONS

- Management of anxiety, panic disorders, premenstrual dysphoric disorders
- Onset 30 minutes, peak 1–2 hours, duration 4–6 hours
- Full therapeutic response takes 2–3 days
- May be taken with food
- May be habit-forming; do not take for longer than 4 months unless directed
- Memory impairment is a sign of long-term use
- Do not stop drug abruptly; may cause seizures
- Drowsiness may worsen at beginning of treatment
- May produce emotional and/or physical dependence
- Rx

. . . .

SIDE EFFECTS

Dizziness, headache
Stimulation, insomnia,
  nervousness

Light-headedness, numbness
Nausea, diarrhea, constipation
Tachycardia, palpitations

NURSING CONSIDERATIONS

- Management of anxiety disorders
- Onset 7–10 days, optimum effect may take 3–4 weeks
- Use caution with activities requiring alertness until response to med is known
- Avoid alcohol, CNS depressants, and large amounts of grapefruit juice
- Use caution when changing positions because fainting may occur, especially in elderly
- Drowsiness may worsen at beginning of treatment
- Rx

CHLORDIAZEPOXIDE
(klor-dye-az-e-<u>pox</u>-ide)

(Librium)

DIAZEPAM
(dye-<u>az</u>-e-pam)

(Valium)

SIDE EFFECTS

Dizziness
Drowsiness
Pain at IM site

Ataxia
Disorientation

NURSING CONSIDERATIONS

- Management of anxiety and treatment of alcohol withdrawal, IBS
- PO: onset 1–2 hours, peak 30 minutes to 4 hours
- IM: onset 15–30 minutes, slow, erratic absorption
- IV: onset 1–5 minutes, duration 15–60 minutes
- Use caution with activities requiring alertness until response to med is known
- Abrupt stop may lead to withdrawal: insomnia, irritability, nervousness, tremors
- Avoid alcohol, CNS depressants
- Tablets may be crushed and taken with food or fluids for ease of swallowing
- Rx; C-IV

• •

SIDE EFFECTS

Drowsiness, fatigue, ataxia
Hypotension
Paradoxic anxiety,
  esp. in elderly

Orthostatic hypotension
Blurred vision

NURSING CONSIDERATIONS

- Treatment of anxiety, acute alcohol withdrawal, seizures; skeletal muscle relaxant; preoperative medication
- PO: may be taken with food, onset 30 minutes
- IM: inject deep, slowly into large muscle mass; onset 15–30 minutes, duration 60–90 minutes, slow and erratic absorption
- IV: into large vein, push doses should not exceed 5 mg/minute, resuscitation equipment available; onset immediate, duration 15 minutes to 1 hour
- Smoking may decrease effectiveness
- Avoid use with alcohol, CNS depressants
- Long-term use withdrawal symptoms: vomiting, sweating, abdominal/ muscle cramps, tremors, and possibly convulsions
- May be habit-forming if used over 4 months
- Rx; C-IV

LORAZEPAM
(lor-<u>a</u>-ze-pam)

(Ativan)

· ·

Mental Health Medications
Antidepressants, SSRIs

CITALOPRAM
(sit-<u>al</u>-oh-pram)

(Celexa)

SIDE EFFECTS

Dizziness, drowsiness
Orthostatic hypotension
Blurred vision

Weakness
Disorientation
Visual disturbance

NURSING CONSIDERATIONS

- Treatment of anxiety, irritability in psychiatric or organic disorders; treatment of insomnia; adjunct in endoscopic procedures; preoperative medication
- PO: onset 30 minutes, peak 1–6 hours
- IM: onset 15–30 minutes, peak 60–90 minutes
- IV: onset 5–15 minutes, peak unknown
- May be taken with food
- May be habit-forming; do not take for longer than 4 months unless directed
- Avoid alcohol, CNS depressants
- Do not stop drug abruptly
- Drowsiness may worsen at beginning of treatment
- Rx

• •

SIDE EFFECTS

Palpitations, tachycardia
Nausea, vomiting, diarrhea
Decreased appetite

Nervousness, insomnia
Drowsiness
Hyponatremia

NURSING CONSIDERATIONS

- Treatment of major depression
- Take in A.M. to avoid insomnia
- Can potentiate effects of digoxin, warfarin, and diazepam
- Avoid use with alcohol, CNS depressants for up to 1 week after end of therapy
- Use caution in potentially hazardous activities
- Avoid changing positions (lying, sitting, standing) rapidly
- Take consistently at same time of day; therapeutic effects in up to 4 weeks
- May increase risk of suicidal thoughts and behavior
- Rx

ESCITALOPRAM OXALATE
(es-sye-<u>tal</u>-oh-pram <u>ox</u>-a-late)

(Lexapro)

• •

FLUOXETINE HCL
(floo-<u>ox</u>-uh-teen)

(Prozac)

SIDE EFFECTS

Effect
Nausea, diarrhea,
  constipation
Insomnia
Fatigue, drowsiness
Decreased libido,
  sexual dysfunction

Increased sweating
Increased appetite,
  heartburn, stomach
  pain
Flulike symptoms,
  runny nose, sneezing
Dry mouth

Dizziness
Labile blood sugar
Hypokalemia
Hyponatremia
Visual disturbances

NURSING CONSIDERATIONS

- Treatment of major depression, anxiety
- Take consistently at same time of day; full therapeutic effect may require 4 weeks
- May require gradual reduction before stopping
- Can potentiate effects of digoxin, warfarin, diazepam
- Use caution in potentially hazardous activities; avoid use with alcohol
- May increase risk of suicidal thoughts or behaviors
- Monitor for SIADH
- Teach patient to avoid aspirin and NSAIDs due to increased bleeding risk
- May cause serotonin syndrome or NMS; monitor for change in mental status, hyperthermia, tachycardia, labile BP, and incoordination
- Rx

• •

SIDE EFFECTS

Palpitations
Nausea, diarrhea, constipation
Decreased appetite with
  significant weight loss
Nervousness, insomnia

Urinary retention
Drowsiness
Rash, pruritus, excessive
  sweating
Fatigue

NURSING CONSIDERATIONS

- Treatment of depression/OCD, bulimia, PMDD
- Used for anorexia, not suicidal or homicidal emotions
- Take consistently at same time of day; full therapeutic effects may require 4 weeks
- Can potentiate effects of digoxin, warfarin, diazepam, NSAIDs, and aspirin
- Avoid use with alcohol, CNS depressants for up to 1 week after end of therapy
- Use caution in potentially hazardous activities
- May increase risk of suicidal thoughts or behavior
- Rx

PAROXETINE HCL
(pa-<u>rox</u>-eh-teen)

(Paxil)

· ·

SERTRALINE HCL
(<u>sir</u>-trah-leen)

(Zoloft)

SIDE EFFECTS

Palpitations
Nausea, vomiting, diarrhea,
  constipation

Hyponatremia
Decreased appetite
Nervousness, insomnia

NURSING CONSIDERATIONS

- Treatment of anxiety, depression, OCD and social anxiety disorder, panic disorder, PTSD
- Take consistently at same time of day; therapeutic effects in up to 4 weeks
- Do not chew or crush
- May increase risk of suicidal thoughts or behavior
- May increase risk for bleeding
- Avoid use with alcohol, CNS depressants for up to 1 week after end of therapy
- Use caution in potentially hazardous activities
- Rx

• •

SIDE EFFECTS

Headache
Dizziness
Tremor
Nausea, diarrhea

Insomnia
Dry mouth
Male sexual dysfunction

NURSING CONSIDERATIONS

- Treatment of depression, OCD, panic disorder with or without agoraphobia, PTSD, PMDD, and social phobia
- Used for anorexia, not suicidal or homicidal emotions
- Take consistently at same time of day; therapeutic effects take up to 4 weeks
- Can potentiate effects of digoxin, warfarin, diazepam, aspirin, and NSAIDs
- Avoid use with alcohol, CNS depressants for up to 1 week after end of therapy; avoid disulfiram
- Use caution in potentially hazardous activities
- May increase risk of suicidal thoughts or behavior
- Rx, Preg Cat C

AMITRIPTYLINE
(a-mee-<u>trip</u>-ti-leen)

· ·

DOXEPIN
(<u>dox</u>-e-pin)

SIDE EFFECTS

Sedation/drowsiness

Blurred vision, dry mouth, diaphoresis

Postural hypotension, palpitations

Nausea, vomiting, diarrhea

Constipation, urinary retention

Increased appetite

Sexual dysfunction

Confusion

Cardiac dysrhythmias

NURSING CONSIDERATIONS

- Treatment of major depression
- Suicide risk high after 10–14 days due to increased energy
- Avoid use with alcohol
- Sunblock required
- Increase fluid intake
- Take dose at bedtime due to sedative effect
- Heavy smokers may require a larger dose
- Use safety precautions with hazardous activity
- Avoid sudden positional changes, partial hypotension
- Blood sugar may be altered; monitor blood sugar in diabetic patients
- Rx

• •

SIDE EFFECTS

Sedation/drowsiness

Blurred vision, dry mouth, diaphoresis

Postural hypotension, palpitations

Nausea, vomiting, diarrhea

Constipation, urinary retention

Anorexia

Sexual dysfunction

NURSING CONSIDERATIONS

- Used in psychoneurotic patients with depression and/or anxiety; hypnotic for insomnia
- Increase fluid intake
- Take dose at bedtime due to sedative effect
- Heavy smokers may require a larger dose
- Avoid use with alcohol
- Suicide risk high after 10–14 day due to increased energy
- Use safety precautions with hazardous activity
- Avoid sudden positional changes
- May cause "sleep" activities such as driving a car, eating, communicating with others
- May worsen depression
- Rx

IMIPRAMINE
(im-<u>ip</u>-ra-meen)

(Tofranil)

NORTRIPTYLINE
(nor-<u>trip</u>-ti-leen)

(Pamelor)

SIDE EFFECTS

Sedation/drowsiness
Dry mouth
Postural hypotension,
  palpitations

Diarrhea
Urinary retention
Anorexia
Confusion

NURSING CONSIDERATIONS

- Used in psychoneurotic patients with depression and anxiety; hypnotic for insomnia
- Drug is dispensed in small amounts at beginning of treatment due to suicide potential
- Full therapeutic effect may take 2–3 weeks
- Use safety precautions with hazardous activity
- Avoid sudden positional changes
- Do not stop abruptly: could cause nausea, malaise, headache
- Avoid alcohol, CNS depressants
- Rx

• •

SIDE EFFECTS

Sedation/drowsiness
Blurred vision, dry mouth,
  diaphoresis
Postural hypotension,
  palpitations

Nausea, vomiting, diarrhea
Constipation, urinary retention
Increased appetite
Sexual dysfunction

NURSING CONSIDERATIONS

- Treatment of major depression
- Increase fluid intake
- Take dose at bedtime due to sedative effect
- Heavy smokers may require a larger dose
- Avoid use with alcohol, CNS depressants
- Suicide risk high after 10–14 days due to increased energy
- Use safety precautions with hazardous activity
- Avoid sudden positional changes, partial hypotension
- Women: avoid use if pregnant, breastfeeding
- Rx

BUPROPION HCL
(byoo-<u>proe</u>-pee-on)
(Wellbutrin, Zyban)

• •

DULOXETINE HCL
(doo-<u>lox</u>-e-teen)
(Cymbalta)

SIDE EFFECTS

Agitation
Nausea, vomiting
Headache
Dry mouth

Tremor
Hypertension
Insomnia
Nervousness

NURSING CONSIDERATIONS

- Treatment of depression and smoking cessation
- If missed dose for depression, take as soon as possible and space remaining doses at not less than 4-hour intervals
- If missed dose for smoking cessation, omit dose
- May require gradual reduction before stopping
- Avoid use with alcohol, CNS depressants for up to 1 week after end of therapy
- Use caution in potentially hazardous activities
- Avoid changing positions (lying, sitting, standing) rapidly
- May increase risk for suicidal thoughts or behavior
- Rx

• •

SIDE EFFECTS

Nausea, vomiting, diar-
  rhea, constipation
Decreased appetite,
  stomach pain
Heartburn
Dry mouth

Increased urination,
  difficulty urinating
Dizziness, headache
Tiredness, weakness,
  drowsiness
Muscle pain or cramps

Increased sweating, night
  sweats
Sexual dysfunction
Uncontrollable shaking
  of a part of the body

NURSING CONSIDERATIONS

- Treatment of depression, anxiety, diabetic neuropathy, and fibromyalgia
- Take the same time daily, once or twice a day for depression; once a day for anxiety, diabetic neuropathy, or fibromyalgia; full therapeutic effects may require 4 weeks
- May require gradual reduction before stopping
- Avoid changing positions (lying, sitting, standing) rapidly
- Avoid use with alcohol
- Use caution in potentially hazardous activities
- May increase risk of suicidal thoughts or behaviors
- Teach patient to avoid aspirin and NSAIDs due to increased bleeding risk
- Monitor BP
- Monitor blood sugar in diabetics; may cause hyperglycemia
- Rx

MIRTAZAPINE

(mer-<u>taz</u>-e-peen)

(Remeron)

. . . .

TRAZODONE

(<u>traz</u>-oh-doan)

SIDE EFFECTS

Drowsiness, dizziness   Dry mouth
Increased appetite, weight gain   Somnolence
Constipation

NURSING CONSIDERATIONS

- Treatment of depression
- Do not use within 14 days of MAOI
- May require gradual reduction before stopping
- Check with clinician before taking OTC cold remedy
- Avoid use with alcohol, CNS depressants for up to 1 week after end of therapy
- Use caution in potentially hazardous activities
- May increase risk for suicidal thoughts or behavior
- Rx

• •

SIDE EFFECTS

Drowsiness   Dizziness   Blurred vision
Hypotension   Priapism   Constipation
Dry mouth   Hyponatremia
Nausea   Somnolence

NURSING CONSIDERATIONS

- Treatment of major depression
- Take with or immediately after meals to lessen GI upset
- If dose missed, take immediately, unless within 4 hours of next dose
- May require gradual reduction before stopping
- Avoid use with alcohol, CNS depressants for up to 1 week after end of therapy
- Use caution in potentially hazardous activities
- Avoid changing positions (lying, sitting, standing) rapidly
- May increase risk of suicidal thoughts or behavior
- Take at same time, preferably at bedtime on empty stomach
- Rx

VENLAFAXINE
(ven-lah-<u>fax</u>-een)

(Effexor, Effexor XR)

• •

HALOPERIDOL
(hal-oh-<u>pair</u>-i-dole)

(Haldol)

SIDE EFFECTS

Abnormal dreams,
insomnia

Anxiety,
nervousness

Dizziness, weakness

Headache

Abdominal pain

Nausea, vomiting,
diarrhea

Anorexia, weight
loss

Sexual dysfunction

Sedation

Mydriasis

Hypertension

Serotonin syndrome

NURSING CONSIDERATIONS

- Treatment of major depression or relapse, generalized anxiety disorder
- Take with food; extended-release tablets should be swallowed whole
- If dose is missed, take immediately unless time for next dose
- May require gradual reduction before stopping if taken over 6 weeks
- Avoid use with alcohol, CNS depressants for up to 1 week after end of therapy
- Use caution in potentially hazardous activities
- Avoid changing positions (lying, sitting, standing) rapidly
- May increase risk of suicidal thoughts or behavior
- May increase risk of GI bleed
- Rx

• •

SIDE EFFECTS

Drowsiness

Dizziness

Hallucinations

Tardive dyskinesia

Tachycardia

Hypotension

Confusion

Hypertension

Dystonia

Hyperpyrexia

Schizophrenia

NURSING CONSIDERATIONS

- Treatment of Tourette syndrome, schizophrenia
- PO concentrate: dilute with water, not coffee or tea
- PO: take with food or full glass of water/milk
- IM: inject slowly, deep into UOQ of buttock; have patient lie down for 30 minutes; do not give IV
- Avoid abrupt withdrawal; discontinue gradually
- Avoid use with alcohol, CNS depressants
- Use caution in potentially hazardous activities
- Avoid changing positions (lying/sitting/standing) rapidly
- Wear protective clothing, sunglasses due to photosensitivity
- Rx

OLANZAPINE

(oh-<u>lan</u>-zuh-peen)

(Zyprexa)

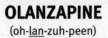

• •

RISPERIDONE

(riss-<u>pair</u>-i-doan)

(Risperdal)

SIDE EFFECTS

Somnolence	Nervousness	Insomnia
Agitation	Joint pain	Increase appetite
Hostility	Dry mouth	and weight gain
Dizziness	Headache	Fatigue
Rhinitis		

NURSING CONSIDERATIONS

- Treatment of schizophrenia and bipolar I disorder
- Has been used successfully in manic episodes associated with bipolar I
- Use caution when rising due to postural hypotension possibility
- Dosage should be managed tightly when established
- Use caution when operating equipment
- Monitor weight
- Monitor blood glucose in diabetic patients; may cause hyperglycemia
- Rx

• •

SIDE EFFECTS

Drowsiness	Constipation	Hyperglycemia
Tardive dyskinesia	Hypersensitivity	Dysphagia
Dizziness	NMS	Priapism

NURSING CONSIDERATIONS

- Treatment of schizophrenia and bipolar I disorder, autistic disorder
- Avoid use with alcohol, CNS depressants
- Use caution in potentially hazardous activities
- Avoid changing positions (lying/sitting/standing) rapidly
- Notify clinician if fever, sore throat, bruising/bleeding, tics/spasms, trembling, shuffling gait
- Avoid strenuous exercise in hot weather
- Check before taking OTC meds
- Monitor blood sugar in diabetic patients
- Rx

QUETIAPINE
(kweh-<u>tie</u>-a-peen)

(Seroquel)

• •

ZIPRASIDONE HCL
(zye-<u>praz</u>-i-doan)

(Geodon)

SIDE EFFECTS

Drowsiness

Dizziness

Hyperglycemia

Hypertension

Dry mouth

Somnolence

Dyspepsia

Weight gain

NURSING CONSIDERATIONS

- Used in treatment of schizophrenia, bipolar I disorder
- Avoid use with alcohol, CNS depressants
- Use caution in potentially hazardous activities
- Avoid changing positions (lying/sitting/standing) rapidly
- Notify clinician if fever, sore throat, bruising/bleeding, tics/ spasms, trembling, shuffling gait
- Avoid strenuous exercise in hot weather
- Check before taking OTC meds
- Monitor blood sugar in diabetic patients
- May increase the risk of suicidal thoughts or behavior
- Monitor BP
- May increase ALT
- Rx

• •

SIDE EFFECTS

Drowsiness

Tardive dyskinesia

Dizziness

Constipation

Somnolence

Abnormal vision

Vomiting

Headache

Hyperglycemia

NMS

NURSING CONSIDERATIONS

- Used in treatment of schizophrenia, bipolar I disorder
- Avoid use with alcohol, CNS depressants
- Use caution in potentially hazardous activities
- Avoid changing positions (lying/sitting/standing) rapidly
- Notify clinician if fever, sore throat, bruising/bleeding, tics/spasms, trembling, shuffling gait
- Avoid strenuous exercise in hot weather
- Check before taking OTC meds
- Women: avoid breastfeeding
- Monitor blood sugar in diabetic patients
- Rx

ARIPIPRAZOLE

(air-i-<u>pip</u>-ray-<u>zole</u>)

(Abilify)

• •

Mental Health Medications
Attention Deficit Disorder Agents

METHYLPHENIDATE HCL

(meth-ill-<u>fen</u>-uh-date)

(Concerta, Ritalin)

SIDE EFFECTS

Headache	Weight gain	Nausea
Agitation	Hyperglycemia	Vomiting
Insomnia	Sedation	Orthostatic
Anxiety	Dyspepsia	hypotension

NURSING CONSIDERATIONS

- Management of schizophrenia (acute and maintenance), bipolar disorder (acute and maintenance); adjunctive therapy for major depressive disorder
- IM: inject deep, slowly into muscle mass; peak 1–3 hours
- PO: can take without regard to food; peak 3–5 hours
- Monitor vital signs, weight, and blood glucose
- Assess for extrapyramidal side effects (less common with atypical antipsychotics)
- Monitor for suicidal ideation
- Rx

• •

SIDE EFFECTS

Headache	Decreased appetite	Nausea
Respiratory	Visual disturbance	Insomnia
infections	Abdominal pain	Restlessness
Hyperhidrosis	Cough	

NURSING CONSIDERATIONS

- Used to treat ADD/ADHD in children over 6 years old, depression in elderly, and narcolepsy
- Concerta is time-released and should be swallowed whole, not chewed
- This prescription cannot be refilled
- Dosage is adjusted in 18-mg increments to a maximum of 54 mg/day
- Contraindicated in patients with anxiety, tension, and glaucoma
- This medication may be habit-forming
- May lower seizure threshold
- Monitor for adverse psychiatric symptoms
- Rx; C-II, Preg Cat C

CARBAMAZEPINE
(kar-ba-<u>maz</u>-e-peen)

(Tegretol, Tegretol XR)

• •

DIVALPROEX SODIUM
(dye-<u>val</u>-proe-ex)

(Depakote)

SIDE EFFECTS

Myelosuppression	Ataxia	Photosensitivity
Dizziness	Diplopia	Nausea, vomiting
Drowsiness	Rash	

NURSING CONSIDERATIONS

- Management of bipolar disorder, seizures, trigeminal neuralgia, diabetic neuropathy
- Take with food or milk to decrease GI upset; tablets (nonextended-release) may be crushed, extended-release capsules may be opened, mixed with juice or soft food
- Avoid driving and other activities requiring alertness for the first 3 days
- Monitor blood levels, CBC regularly, especially during first 2 months; periodic eye exams
- Urine may turn pink to brown
- Avoid abrupt withdrawal; discontinue gradually
- Avoid use with alcohol, CNS depressants
- Monitor for hepatic reactions
- Monitor thyroid function
- Monitor for suicidal thoughts or behavior
- Patient should wear medical information tag
- Rx

• •

SIDE EFFECTS

Sedation, drowsiness, dizziness	Prolonged bleeding time
Mental status and behavioral changes	Teratogenicity
	Pancreatitis
Nausea, vomiting, constipation, diarrhea, heartburn	Hepatotoxicity

NURSING CONSIDERATIONS

- Management of seizures, manic episodes assoc. with bipolar disorder (delayed-release only), migraine prophylaxis (delayed- and extended-release only)
- Take with or immediately after meals to lessen GI upset
- Swallow tablets or capsules whole (no crushing, chewing)
- Delayed-release products: peak blood level 3–5 hours, duration 12–24 hours
- Extended-release products: peak blood level 7–14 hours, duration 24 hours
- Avoid abrupt withdrawal after long-term use; discontinue gradually to prevent convulsions
- Monitor blood levels, platelets, bleeding time, and liver function tests
- Monitor for suicidal thoughts or behavior
- Wear medical information tag
- Rx

LITHIUM
(li-thee-um)

(Lithobid)

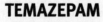

TEMAZEPAM
(tem-az-eh-pam)

(Restoril)

SIDE EFFECTS

Dizziness

Impaired vision

Fine hand tremors

Reversible leukocytosis

Signs of intoxication: vomiting, diarrhea, drowsiness, muscular weakness, ataxia

NURSING CONSIDERATIONS

- Controls manic episodes in manic-depressive individuals; mood stabilizer
- Use caution in potentially hazardous activities
- Check serum levels 2 times weekly during treatment, q 2–3 months on maintenance; draw blood in A.M. prior to dose
- Target serum levels: treatment = 0.5 to 1.5 mEq/L, maintenance = 0.6–1.2 mEq/L
- GI symptoms reduced if taken with meals
- Onset of therapeutic effects in 1–2 weeks
- Diabetics: closely monitor blood/urine glucose
- Dose reduced during depressive stages of illness
- Encourage 10–12 glasses water/day and adequate salt intake (6–10 g/day)
- Avoid caffeine, increased exercise, saunas
- Rx

• •

SIDE EFFECTS

Drowsiness

Dizziness

Lethargy

Weakness

Euphoria

Anorexia

Headache

Fatigue

NURSING CONSIDERATIONS

- Used for short-term (7–10 days) treatment of insomnia
- Should be avoided in patients under the age of 18
- Avoid alcohol while taking this drug
- Not intended for use for more than 10 days
- When used with CNS depressants, the CNS depression is increased
- "Sleep driving" may occur, especially if taken with alcohol or CNS depressants
- Rx; C-IV

ZALEPLON
(zall-e-plon)

(Sonata)

• •

ZOLPIDEM TARTRATE
(zol-pi-dem)

(Ambien)

SIDE EFFECTS

Headache
Myalgia
Dizziness

Asthenia
Dyspepsia
Eye pain

NURSING CONSIDERATIONS

- Used in short-term insomnia treatment
- Zaleplon does not prolong sleep time or decrease awakenings
- Elderly patients generally benefit the most
- Because of rapid onset, patients should take immediately before bedtime
- Avoid alcohol while using this medication
- May be habit-forming
- "Sleep driving" may occur
- Rx; C-IV

• •

SIDE EFFECTS

Headache
Drowsiness
Influenza-like symptoms

Dizziness
Nausea
"Drugged" feeling

NURSING CONSIDERATIONS

- Short-term treatment of insomnia
- Dosage may need to be adjusted down if patient is using a CNS depressant to avoid an addictive effect
- Side effects increase with prolonged usage
- May cause "sleep driving"
- May worsen depression
- Monitor for suicidal thoughts or behavior
- Rx

ALLOPURINOL
(al-oh-<u>pure</u>-i-nole)

(Aloprim, Zyloprim)

• •

Musculoskeletal Medications
Antigout Agents

COLCHICINE
(<u>kol</u>-chi-seen)

(Colcrys)

SIDE EFFECTS

GI upset

Rash

Headache, drowsiness

NURSING CONSIDERATIONS

- Treatment of gout, uric acid neuropathy, uric acid stone formation
- Encourage 10–12 glasses water/day
- Check CBC and renal function tests
- Take with food; don't take vitamin C or iron
- Initial therapy can increase attacks of gout
- Avoid use of alcohol, eating organ meats, gravy, legumes
- Full therapeutic effect may require several months
- Management of patients with leukemia, lymphoma who are receiving chemotherapy that may increase uric acid
- Monitor liver function tests
- Rx

• •

SIDE EFFECTS

Nausea, vomiting, diarrhea

Agranulocytosis

Sign of toxicity: abdominal cramp

Pharyngolaryngeal pain

NURSING CONSIDERATIONS

- Treatment and prevention of acute gout attacks, familial Mediterranean fever
- Has analgesic, anti-inflammatory effects
- May be taken without regard to meals
- IV: slowly; do not administer IM/subQ
- Encourage 10–12 glasses water/day
- Avoid use of alcohol, eating organ meats, gravy, legumes
- Always carry medication to treat acute attacks
- Grapefruit and grapefruit juice should not be consumed
- Rx

PROBENECID

(proe-<u>ben</u>-e-sid)

(Probalan)

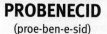

DICLOFENAC NA

(dye-<u>kloe</u>-fen-ak)

(Voltaren)

SIDE EFFECTS

Nausea
Sore gums, anorexia
Hypersensitivity

Skin rash
Hemolytic anemia

NURSING CONSIDERATIONS

- Treatment of hyperuricemia associated with gout, gouty arthritis
- May also be used with penicillin to elevate and prolong plasma of penicillin for gonococcal infection
- Give with milk, food, and antacids
- Encourage 8–10 glasses water/day
- Check BUN, renal function tests
- Avoid use of alcohol, eating organ meats, gravy, legumes
- Avoid aspirin-containing products; may take acetaminophen
- Rx

• •

SIDE EFFECTS

Dizziness
Blood dyscrasias
Headache
Nephrotoxicity

Hypersensitivity
GI distress, bleeding, or ulcer
Rash

NURSING CONSIDERATIONS

- Used in arthritic conditions, dysmenorrhea
- Ophthalmic: reduce inflammation after cataract extraction
- PO: take with full glass of water and food and remain upright for 30 minutes
- If dose missed, take within 2 hours
- Use sunscreen to prevent photosensitivity
- May increase risk of cardiovascular thrombotic events
- Possible cross-allergy with aspirin and other NSAIDs
- May increase risk of elevated liver tests
- Rx

ETODOLAC
(ee-<u>toe</u>-doe-lak)

• •

IBUPROFEN
(eye-byoo-<u>proe</u>-fen)
(Advil, Motrin IB)

SIDE EFFECTS

Nephrotoxicity
Nausea
Blood dyscrasias
Anorexia

Dizziness
Hypertension
Hypersensitivity

NURSING CONSIDERATIONS

- Reduces pain of osteoarthritis, rheumatoid arthritis
- Monitor for signs of toxicity: blurred vision, ringing or roaring in ears
- Full therapeutic effect may take up to 1 month
- Avoid concurrent use of ASA, NSAIDs, acetaminophen, alcohol
- May increase risk of cardiovascular thrombotic events
- May increase risk of GI bleeding or ulcer
- May cause false positive for urinary bilirubin
- May cause false positive for ketones in urine
- Rx

• •

SIDE EFFECTS

Nausea, vomiting, diarrhea,
  constipation
Headache, dizziness
Fluid retention

GI bleeding
Hives
Rash

NURSING CONSIDERATIONS

- Treatment of rheumatoid arthritis/osteoarthritis; relief of mild/moderate pain; antipyretic
- Take with milk or food
- Use cautiously with aspirin allergy
- Monitor for visual disturbances, tinnitus
- Monitor for increased weight gain, edema, fever, hematuria, arthralgia
- Avoid alcohol
- OTC, Rx

INDOMETHACIN

(in-doe-<u>meth</u>-a-sin)

(Indocin)

• •

NAPROXEN NA

(na-<u>prox</u>-en)

(Aleve, Anaprox, Naprosyn)

SIDE EFFECTS

Peptic ulcer
Dizziness
Bone marrow depression
Hypersensitivity

Blurred vision
Tinnitus
Hypertension
Drowsiness

NURSING CONSIDERATIONS

- Treatment of rheumatoid arthritis/osteoarthritis, acute gout, acute painful shoulder
- PO: take with food/milk, encourage upright position for 15–30 minutes
- Use caution with potentially hazardous activities
- Avoid use with alcohol, aspirin, other NSAIDs
- Observe for bleeding problems
- May increase risk for cardiovascular thrombotic events
- Monitor for weight gain
- Rx

• •

SIDE EFFECTS

Nausea
Dizziness
Headache

Asthma
GI bleeding
Hives

NURSING CONSIDERATIONS

- For mild to moderate pain; treatment of arthritis, primary dysmenorrhea
- PO: with food to decrease GI upset; on empty stomach to increase absorption
- Monitor for signs of toxicity: blurred vision, ringing or roaring in ears
- Full therapeutic effect may take up to 1 month
- Avoid concurrent use of ASA, steroids, alcohol
- Monitor for melena, weight gain, arthralgia, hematuria
- OTC, Rx

PIROXICAM
(peer-<u>ox</u>-i-kam)

(Feldene)

SALSALATE
(<u>sal</u>-sah-late)

(Disalcid)

SIDE EFFECTS

Drowsiness
Headache
Hypertension

Hypersensitivity
GI disturbances, bleeding or
  ulcer

NURSING CONSIDERATIONS

- For mild to moderate pain, osteoarthritis, rheumatoid arthritis
- PO: with food to decrease GI upset; on empty stomach to increase absorption
- Take at same time every day
- Monitor for signs of toxicity: blurred vision, ringing or roaring in ears, jaundice
- Full therapeutic effect may take up to 1 month
- Avoid concurrent use of ASA, OTC meds, alcohol
- May increase risk of cardiovascular thrombotic events
- Rx

• •

SIDE EFFECTS

Nausea, vomiting
GI bleeding
Vertigo

Heartburn
Rash
Tinnitus

NURSING CONSIDERATIONS

- For mild to moderate pain, rheumatoid arthritis, and osteoarthritis
- PO: can be crushed or taken whole
- PO: take with food or milk to decrease GI upset
- Full therapeutic effect may take 2 weeks
- Read label on OTC meds, may contain ASA
- Monitor for signs of toxicity: changes in liver, kidney, eye, ear functions
- Rx

BACLOFEN
(<u>bak</u>-loe-fen)

(Lioresal)

• •

CARISOPRODOL
(kar-eye-soe-<u>proe</u>-dole)

(Soma)

SIDE EFFECTS

Drowsiness
Dizziness
Weakness, fatigue
Confusion

Nausea, vomiting
Headache
Seizures

NURSING CONSIDERATIONS

- Used to reduce spasticity in multiple sclerosis, spinal cord injury, flexor spasms, and muscular rigidity
- Take with food
- Avoid alcohol, CNS depressants
- Increased risk of seizures in patients with seizure disorder
- Withdraw gradually over 1 to 2 weeks, unless severe adverse reactions; D/C may cause hallucinations, tachycardia, or rebound spasticity
- Monitor for symptoms of sensitivity: fever, skin eruptions, respiratory distress
- May elevate blood sugar, monitor blood sugar in diabetic patients
- Rx

• •

SIDE EFFECTS

Drowsiness
Light-headedness
Headache

Dizziness
Nausea

NURSING CONSIDERATIONS

- Relief of pain, stiffness associated with musculoskeletal conditions
- PO: onset 30 minutes, peak 4 hours, duration 4–6 hours
- Avoid alcohol, CNS depressants, including OTC cold or allergy meds
- Avoid activities requiring alertness until effects of medication are known
- May cause dependence; this is not a controlled substance
- Rx

CYCLOBENZAPRINE
(sye-kloe-<u>ben</u>-za-preen)

(Flexeril)

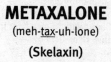

METAXALONE
(meh-<u>tax</u>-uh-lone)

(Skelaxin)

SIDE EFFECTS

Drowsiness
Dizziness
Fatigue

Dry mouth
Constipation
Headache

NURSING CONSIDERATIONS

- Relieves muscle spasms from acute conditions
- Avoid alcohol, CNS depressants, including OTC cold or allergy meds
- Avoid activities requiring alertness until effects of medication are known
- Rx

• •

SIDE EFFECTS

Drowsiness
Gastrointestinal pains
Nervousness

Dizziness
Headache
Irritability

NURSING CONSIDERATIONS

- Used to relieve painful musculoskeletal injuries
- Should be an adjunct to rest and physical therapy
- Avoid alcohol while using this drug
- Use caution when operating machinery
- Use cautiously in patients with known liver impairment
- May cause false positive Benedict's test
- Rx

METHOCARBAMOL
(meth-oh-<u>kar</u>-ba-mole)

(Robaxin)

· ·

BENZTROPINE
(<u>benz</u>-troe-peen)

(Cogentin)

SIDE EFFECTS

Drowsiness
Light-headedness

Dizziness
Nausea

NURSING CONSIDERATIONS

- Relieves muscle spasms from acute conditions, tetanus management
- IM: inject deep into UOQ of buttock, rotate sites
- NG tube: crush tablets into fluid
- PO: take with food or milk
- Metallic taste may develop
- Urine may turn green, black, or brown
- Avoid alcohol, CNS depressants, including OTC cold or allergy meds
- Avoid activities requiring alertness until effects of medication are known
- Monitor IV sites carefully for extravasation
- Rx

• •

SIDE EFFECTS

Dry mouth
Constipation
Anhidrosis

Weakness
Tardive dyskinesia

NURSING CONSIDERATIONS

- Treatment of Parkinson symptoms, EPS associated with neuroleptic drugs, acute dystonic reactions
- IM/IV: onset 15 minutes, duration 6–10 hours
- PO: onset 1 hour, duration 6–10 hours
- Tablets may be crushed and mixed with food
- Taper med over a week, or withdrawal symptoms: EPS, tremors, insomnia, tachycardia, restlessness
- Avoid hazardous activities until stabilized on med
- Change positions slowly
- Avoid alcohol, antihistamines unless directed by clinician
- Antidote is physostigmine
- Rx

CAFFEINE/ERGOTAMINE
(er-got-a-meen)

(Cafergot)

· ·

CARBIDOPA/LEVODOPA
(kar-bih-doe-pa/leev-oe-doe-pa)

(Sinemet)

SIDE EFFECTS

Headache
Tremors, convulsions
Blood vessel contraction, with decreased circulation, esp. in limbs

Toxic ergotism: nausea, vomiting, diarrhea, dizziness, headache, mental confusion

NURSING CONSIDERATIONS

- Treatment of vascular headache
- Take at onset of pain/during prodromal stage to abort headache
- Lie down in darkened quiet room for several hours
- Rx

. . . .

SIDE EFFECTS

Twitching
Headache, dizziness
Mental changes: confusion, agitation, mood alterations

Dark urine/sweat
Cardiac arrhythmias

NURSING CONSIDERATIONS

- Treatment for Parkinson disease and syndrome
- Replacement dopaminergic agent
- Take with food; decreased effect with liver, pork, wheat germ, and vitamin B6
- Full therapeutic effect may take several months
- Change positions slowly
- Monitor for melanoma
- May cause dark color in saliva, urine, or sweat
- May increase liver function test results
- May cause false positive for urine ketones
- Rx

DONEPEZIL

(doe-<u>nep</u>-uh-zill)

(Aricept)

- -

GALANTAMINE, RIVASTIGMINE

(ga-<u>lan</u>-ta-meen, ri-va-<u>stig</u>-meen)

(Razadyne, Exelon)

SIDE EFFECTS

Nausea, vomiting, diarrhea
Headache, dizziness
Fatigue
Twitching
Cardiac arrhythmias
Insomnia

Seizures
Rash
Dark urine/sweat
Mental changes: confusion,
    agitation, mood alterations

NURSING CONSIDERATIONS

- Used in treatment of all stages of Alzheimer's disease
- Drug does not cure, but stabilizes or relieves symptoms
- Take at regular intervals
- Take between meals or may be given with meals to decrease GI upset
- May increase BUN, SGOT, GPT
- Rx

• •

SIDE EFFECTS

Nausea
Vomiting
Loss of appetite

Increased frequency of bowel movements

NURSING CONSIDERATIONS

- Treatment of dementia associated with mild to moderate Alzheimer's disease
- Galantamine and rivastigmine are cholinesterase inhibitors, which increase acetylcholine in the brain, potentially reducing symptoms of dementia
- Neither drug alters the underlying disease process
- Use with caution in patients with liver, bladder, or renal disease
- Rx

LISDEXAMFETAMINE DIMESYLATE
(lis-dex-am-<u>fet</u>-a-meen dye-<u>mes</u>-i-late)

(Vyvanse)

· ·

MEMANTINE HCL
(<u>mem</u>-an-teen)

(Namenda XR)

Side Effects

Insomnia
Irritability
Decreased appetite

Dry mouth
Upper abdominal pain

Nursing Considerations

- Treatment of attention-deficit hyperactivity disorder (ADHD)
- For individuals age 6 years through adult; effects have not been studied in the elderly
- Interrupt therapy occasionally to determine if there is recurrence of behavioral symptoms sufficient to require continued therapy
- Children and adolescents: sudden death has been reported in patients with structural cardiac abnormalities or other serious heart problems taking CNS stimulant treatment at usual doses
- Adults: sudden death, stroke, and MI have occurred in adults taking stimulant drugs in ADHD doses
- Rx

. . . .

Side Effects

Headache
Constipation

Confusion
Dizziness

Nursing Considerations

- Treatment of dementia in moderate to severe Alzheimer's disease
- Unlike other Alzheimer's meds, memantine is not a cholinesterase inhibitor; regulates the activity of glutamate, a chemical messenger involved in learning and memory
- Does not alter underlying disease process
- Use with caution in patients with liver, bladder, or renal disease
- Capsules can be opened and contents sprinkled on applesauce for patients who have difficulty swallowing pills
- Rx

METHYLPHENIDATE
(meth-ill-<u>fen</u>-i-date)

(Concerta, Ritalin)

• •

SELEGILINE
(se-<u>leh</u>-ji-leen)

(Eldepryl)

SIDE EFFECTS

Hyperactivity, insomnia
Restlessness
Talkativeness

Palpitations, tachycardia
Hyperhidrosis
Anorexia

Visual disturbance
Nausea
Abdominal pain
Cough

NURSING CONSIDERATIONS

- Management of ADHD, narcolepsy, depression in the elderly
- Onset 30 minutes, duration 4–6 hours
- Take at least 6 hours before bedtime (regular-release) or 10 hours before bedtime (sustained-release, extended-release)
- Taper med over several weeks or depression, increased sleeping, lethargy will occur
- Avoid hazardous activities until stabilized on med
- Decrease caffeine consumption (coffee, tea, cola, chocolate) to decrease irritability
- Monitor for adverse psychiatric symptoms
- May lower seizure threshold
- Rx; C-II

• •

SIDE EFFECTS

Dizziness
Cardiac dysrhythmias
Rhinitis

Nausea
Pain
Headache
Back pain

Dyspepsia
Insomnia

NURSING CONSIDERATIONS

- Used in management of Parkinson disease with levodopa/carbidopa
- Do not use with tricyclics or opioids; do not use with meperidine
- Monitor for signs of toxicity: twitching, eye spasms
- Do not stop abruptly; parkinsonian crisis may occur
- Avoid foods high in tyramine: cheese, pickled products, alcohol, large amounts of caffeine
- Monitor for melanoma
- Monitor for intense urges (gambling, sexual)
- Rx

ZOLMITRIPTAN
(zole-mih-<u>trip</u>-tan)

(Zomig)

• •

DORZOLAMIDE HCL
(dor-<u>zoh</u>-la-mide)

(Trusopt)

SIDE EFFECTS

Weakness, neck stiffness
Tingling, hot sensation,
  burning, feeling of pressure,
  tightness

Numbness, dizziness, sedation
Hypertension
Dyspepsia
Dry mouth

NURSING CONSIDERATIONS

- Used for treatment of acute migraine with or without aura
- Take as soon as symptoms occur
- PO: tablet may be split
- Avoid foods high in tyramine: cheese, pickled products, alcohol, large amounts of caffeine
- May cause serotonin syndrome when used with antidepression medication
- Rx

• •

SIDE EFFECTS

Ocular burning, stinging,
  discomfort
Blurred vision, tearing, or
  dryness

Photophobia
Bitter taste in mouth

NURSING CONSIDERATIONS

- Treatment of glaucoma and ocular hypertension
- Wash hands before and after instillation
- Do not touch tip of dropper to eye or body
- Do not wear contact lens during instillation
- Drug is a sulfonamide; although given topically, it can be absorbed systemically
- Stop med if eye inflammation or eyelid reactions occur
- Rx

DORZOLAMIDE/TIMOLOL

(dor-<u>zoh</u>-la-mide/<u>tye</u>-moe-lole)

(Cosopt)

• •

TRAVOPROST

(<u>trav</u>-oh-prahst)

(Travatan)

SIDE EFFECTS

Ocular burning, stinging, discomfort

Blurred vision, tearing, or dryness

Photophobia

Bitter taste in mouth

NURSING CONSIDERATIONS

- Treatment of glaucoma and ocular hypertension
- Place pressure on tear ducts for 1 minute
- Wash hands before and after instillation
- Do not touch drug container to eye or body
- Do not wear contact lens during instillation
- Drug contains sulfonamide; although given topically, it can be absorbed systemically
- Stop if eye inflammation or eyelid reactions
- Rx

• •

SIDE EFFECTS

Effect

Ocular hyperemia

Decreased visual acuity

Eye discomfort or pain

Foreign-body sensation

Eye pruritus

NURSING CONSIDERATIONS

- Treatment of glaucoma and ocular hypertension for patients who can't tolerate or respond inadequately to other IOP-lowering drugs
- Place pressure on tear ducts for 1 minute
- Wash hands before and after instillation
- Do not touch tip of dropper to eye or body
- Potential for increased brown pigmentation of iris, eyelid skin darkening, changes in eyelashes; important if only one eye is being treated
- Stop if eye inflammation or eyelid reactions
- Remove contact lens to give med; can reinsert in 15 minutes
- Discard med 6 months after opening
- Rx

LEVOBUNOLOL
(lee-voe-<u>byoo</u>-no-lole)

(AK-Beta, Betagan)

• •

TIMOLOL
(<u>tim</u>-oh-lole)

(Timoptic, Betimol solution)

SIDE EFFECTS

Hypotension
Transient eye stinging and
  burning

Asthma attacks in patients with
  history of asthma
Bradycardia

NURSING CONSIDERATIONS

- Treatment of glaucoma and ocular hypertension
- Place pressure on tear ducts for 1 minute
- Wash hands before and after instillation
- Do not touch tip of dropper to eye or body
- Drug is a beta blocker
- Although given topically, it can be absorbed systemically
- Report shortness of breath, chest pain, or heart irregularity
- Monitor diabetic patients for hypoglycemia
- Wear medical information tag
- Rx

• •

SIDE EFFECTS

Fatigue
Weakness
Hypotension

Burning and stinging of eye
Bradycardia

NURSING CONSIDERATIONS

- Treatment of glaucoma and ocular hypertension
- Place pressure on tear ducts for 1 minute
- Wash hands before and after instillation
- Do not touch drug container to eye or body
- Monitor for hypoglycemia in diabetic patients
- Rx

BRIMONIDINE TARTRATE
(brih-<u>moh</u>-nih-deen)

(Alphagan P)

• •

CROMOLYN NA
(<u>kroe</u>-moe-lin)

(Opticrom)

SIDE EFFECTS

Ocular hyperemia
Allergic conjunctivitis
Pruritus

Fatigue
Hypertension
Visual disturbance

NURSING CONSIDERATIONS

- Treatment of glaucoma and ocular hypertension
- Wait 15 minutes after use to wear soft contact lens
- Use caution with hazardous activities due to decreased mental alertness
- Avoid alcohol
- Monitor intraocular pressure because may reverse after 1 month of therapy
- Rx

• •

SIDE EFFECTS

Ocular irritation
Hypersensitivity

NURSING CONSIDERATIONS

- Used in treatment of conjunctivitis, keratitis
- Wash hands before and after instillation
- Do not touch tip of dropper to eye or body
- Do not wear soft contact lens while using this medication
- Rx

ANTIPYRINE/BENZOCAINE/ GLYCERIN OTIC SOLUTION
(an-tee-<u>pye</u>-reen/<u>ben</u>-zoe-kane/<u>gli</u>-sa-rin <u>oh</u>-tik)

(Auralgan)

• •

HYDROCORTISONE/NEOMYCIN/ POLYMYXIN OTIC
(hye-droe-<u>kor</u>-tir-sone/nee-ch-<u>mye</u>-sin/pol-i-<u>mix</u>-in)

(Cortisporin)

SIDE EFFECTS
Hypersensitivity

NURSING CONSIDERATIONS
- Otic analgesic inflammation
- Suspension: shake well (also comes in solution)
- Can warm up with hands for patient's comfort
- Warn patient not to touch ear with dropper
- Warn patient that drug is for use in ears only
- Do not get in eyes, nose, or mouth
- May place cotton plug moistened with Auralgan in ear canal
- Do not rinse dropper
- Rx

• •

SIDE EFFECTS
Hypersensitivity	Dryness
Burning	Skin atrophy

NURSING CONSIDERATIONS
- Otic analgesic and antibiotic for treatment of bacterial infections of external auditory canal
- Warn patient not to touch ear with dropper
- Explain drug is for use in ears only
- Possible cross allergy with kanamycin, paromomycin, streptomycin, and gentamicin
- Rx

CROMOLYN SODIUM INHALER
(<u>kroe</u>-moe-lin)

(Intal)

. . . .

MONTELUKAST
(mon-te-<u>lew</u>-kast)

(Singulair)

SIDE EFFECTS

Bronchospasm   Dizziness
Cough, wheeze   Nausea

NURSING CONSIDERATIONS

- Prophylactic management of bronchial asthma
- Notify clinician of wheezing, respiratory distress
- Do not use for acute asthma attacks
- Full therapeutic effect may take several weeks
- Rx

• •

SIDE EFFECTS

Dizziness   Pharyngitis   Runny nose
Headache   Cough   Sinusitis
URI   GI upset
Fever   Otitis media

NURSING CONSIDERATIONS

- Prophylaxis and treatment of chronic asthma and allergic rhinitis
- Do not use to treat acute symptoms; use a rapid-acting bronchodilator
- Notify clinician of wheezing, respiratory distress
- Full therapeutic effect may take several weeks
- May increase risk of neuropsychiatric events including hallucination, aggression, anxiousness, suicidal behavior and thinking, and tremor
- Rx

THEOPHYLLINE
(thee-<u>off</u>-i-lin)

• •

TIOTROPIUM
(tye-oh-<u>troe</u>-pee-um)
(Spiriva, Handihaler)

SIDE EFFECTS

Restlessness	Dizziness	Headache
Palpitations, sinus tachycardia	Anorexia	Insomnia
	Vomiting	

NURSING CONSIDERATIONS

- Treatment of bronchial asthma, bronchospasm of COPD, chronic bronchitis, emphysema
- PO: peak 2 hours; take with full glass of water; best on empty stomach
- Solution: peak 1 hour
- Check all OTC and other meds for ephedrine before taking with this med
- Avoid alcohol, caffeine, smoking
- Avoid activities requiring alertness until response to med is known
- Contact clinician if toxicity: nausea, vomiting, anxiety, insomnia, convulsions
- Drink 8–10 glasses of fluid per day
- Do not crush enteric-coated SR preparations, swallow whole
- Rx

• •

SIDE EFFECTS

Xerostomia	Pharyngitis
Oral thrush	Headache
Rhinitis	Cough

NURSING CONSIDERATIONS

- Maintenance treatment of COPD
- Take once daily
- Oral inhalation: onset 30 minutes, peak 2 hours, duration 24 hours
- Teach how to correctly use inhaler: insert dry powder capsule into inhaler device just before inhalation; do not swallow capsules; rinse mouth with water after inhalation (decreases side effects)
- Do not use as a rescue inhaler (delayed onset, long duration of action)
- Rx

BENZONATATE
(ben-<u>zoe</u>-na-tate)

(Tessalon)

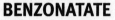

HYDROCODONE
(hye-droe-<u>koe</u>-done)

(Hycodan, with acetaminophen Vicodin)

SIDE EFFECTS

Dizziness

Drowsiness

Rash

Sedation headache

Nausea

NURSING CONSIDERATIONS

- Treatment of nonproductive cough
- PO: onset 15–20 minutes, duration 3–8 hours
- Capsules should be swallowed whole; do not chew, because release of med may cause local anesthetic effect and choking
- Additive CNS depression may occur with antihistamines, alcohol, opioids, and sedative/hypnotics
- Avoid activities requiring alertness until response to med is known
- Contact clinician if signs of overdose: convulsions, trembling, restlessness
- Check lungs regularly
- Rx

• •

SIDE EFFECTS

Nausea, vomiting

Anorexia

Circulatory and respiratory depression

Constipation

Drowsiness

NURSING CONSIDERATIONS

- Treatment of hyperactive and nonproductive cough, mild pain relief
- Physical dependency may result when used for extended periods
- Withdrawal symptoms may occur: nausea, vomiting, cramps, fever, faintness, anorexia
- Avoid CNS depressants
- Onset 10–20 minutes, duration 4–6 hours
- Do not perform potentially dangerous tasks after taking medication
- Rx

IPRATROPIUM BROMIDE
(eye-pra-<u>troe</u>-pee-um)

(Atrovent)

• •

Respiratory Medications
Bronchodilators, Sympathomimetic

ALBUTEROL SULFATE
(al-<u>byoo</u>-ter-ol)

(Proventil-HFA, ProAir HFA)

SIDE EFFECTS

Nervousness
Tremors
Dry mouth
Palpitations
URI

Epistaxis (nosebleed)
Rhinitis
Pharyngitis
Angioedema

NURSING CONSIDERATIONS

- Treatment of bronchospasm associated with COPD, rhinorrhea, rhinitis
- Not for acute bronchospasm needing rapid response
- Teach use of metered dose inhaler: inhale, hold breath, exhale slowly
- Don't mix in nebulizer with cromolyn sodium
- Assess for hypersensitivity, including soy products, atropine, peanuts
- Encourage 10–12 glasses water/day
- Avoid OTC cough/hayfever medications
- Use caution with hazardous activities
- Rx

• •

SIDE EFFECTS

Tremors
Headache
Hyperactivity
Tachycardia
Nausea, vomiting

URI
Rhinitis
Hypersensitivity
GI upset

NURSING CONSIDERATIONS

- Treatment of bronchial asthma, reversible bronchospasm, prevention of exercise-induced asthma
- Teach patient how to correctly use inhaler
- Monitor for toxicity
- PO: take with food to decrease GI upset; may crush tablets
- Teach patient how to take radial pulse
- Rx

SALMETEROL
(sal-<u>meh</u>-teh-role)

(Serevent)

• •

TERBUTALINE SULFATE
(ter-<u>byoo</u>-ta-leen)

SIDE EFFECTS

Headache	Throat irritation
Hypersensitivity	Myalgia
URI	Nausea, vomiting

NURSING CONSIDERATIONS

- Long-term control of asthma, prevention of exercise-induced asthma, prevention of bronchospasm in COPD
- Do not use to treat acute symptoms; do not as a use a rapid-acting bronchodilator
- Contact clinician if difficulty breathing, if more inhalations are needed of rapid-acting bronchodilator, using more than 4 inhalations of a rapid-acting bronchodilator for 2 or more consecutive days, or more than one canister in 8 weeks
- Teach patient inhaler setup and use
- Avoid exposure to chickenpox and measles
- Rx

. . . .

SIDE EFFECTS

Nervousness	Chest pains
Restlessness	Rapid pulse
Tremor	Headache
Palpations	

NURSING CONSIDERATIONS

- Management of asthma or COPD and bronchospasm
- Inhalation and subQ used for short-term control; PO as long-term
- PO: take with food to decrease GI upset
- Tablets may be crushed and mixed with food or fluids
- subQ: give injections in lateral deltoid
- Contact clinician if unrelieved shortness of breath
- Teach patient how to take radial pulse
- Rx

GUAIFENESIN
(gwye-<u>fen</u>-e-sin)

(Robitussin, Mucinex, Mytussin)

· ·

CROMOLYN SODIUM
(<u>kroe</u>-moe-lin)

(NasalCrom)

SIDE EFFECTS
Nausea

NURSING CONSIDERATIONS
- Helps loosen mucous and bronchial secretions to make coughs more productive
- PO: onset 30 minutes, duration 4–6 hours
- PO extended-release: duration 12 hours
- Do not crush pills
- Take with full glass of water
- OTC, Rx

. . . .

SIDE EFFECTS
Nasal burning and irritation   Epistaxis (nosebleed)
Headache   Postnasal drip
Bad taste

NURSING CONSIDERATIONS
- Prophylaxis and treatment of allergic rhinitis
- Full therapeutic effect may take several weeks
- Rx

DISULFIRAM

(dye-<u>sul</u>-fih-ram)

(Antabuse)

• •

MINOXIDIL

(mi-<u>nox</u>-i-dill)

(topical Rogaine)

SIDE EFFECTS

In the absence of alcohol: drowsiness, headache, restlessness, fatigue
In the presence of alcohol: flushing, chest pain, heart arrhythmias,
  hypotension, seizures, throbbing in head and neck, sweating

NURSING CONSIDERATIONS

- Used for treatment of chronic alcoholism by causing severe
  hypersensitivity
- Onset may be delayed up to 12 hours; single dose may be effective
  for 1–2 weeks
- Never give without patient's knowledge
- Avoid alcohol in any form: in foods, sauces, or other meds, such
  as cough syrups or tonics
- Avoid vinegar, paregoric, skin products, liniments, or lotions
  containing alcohol
- Do not begin treatment for at least 12 hours after drinking alcohol
- Wear medical information tag
- Rx

• •

SIDE EFFECTS

Edema   Rash
Increase in body hair

NURSING CONSIDERATIONS

- Topical application (Rogaine) approved to promote hair growth
  in men and women
- Check for weight gain, edema
- Do not use on children or infants
- Avoid contact with eyes, mucous membranes, or sensitive skin
  areas
- OTC, Rx

CARBONYL IRON
(<u>kar</u>-bo-nill)

• •

FERRIC GLUCONATE COMPLEX
(Ferrlecit)

SIDE EFFECTS

Nausea, constipation   Black or discolored stools
Epigastric pain

NURSING CONSIDERATIONS

- Treatment of iron deficiency anemia, prophylaxis for iron deficiency in pregnancy
- Contains 100% elemental iron
- Keep upright for 15–30 minutes to avoid esophageal corrosion, take 1 hour before bedtime
- Stools will become black or dark green
- Notify clinician if stools are tarry or blood-streaked; indicates GI bleeding
- Do not substitute one iron salt for another because iron content differs
- Do not take within 1 hour before or 2 hours after antacids, eggs, whole-grain bread or cereal, milk, coffee, or tea
- Rx

• •

SIDE EFFECTS

Nausea, constipation	Chest pain
Epigastric pain	Fatigue
Black or discolored stools	Cramps
Hypersensitivity	Hypotension
Injection site reaction	Itching

NURSING CONSIDERATIONS

- Treatment of iron deficiency anemia in dialysis patients, given IV
- Onset 4 days, peak 1–2 weeks
- Stools will become black or dark green
- Notify clinician if stools are tarry or blood-streaked; indicates GI bleeding
- Do not mix with other medication
- Only mix with 0.9% sodium chloride
- Rx

FERROUS FUMARATE
(Femiron, Feostat)

• •

FERROUS GLUCONATE
(Fergon)

SIDE EFFECTS

Nausea, constipation   Black or discolored stools
Epigastric pain

NURSING CONSIDERATIONS

- Treatment of iron deficiency anemia, prophylaxis for iron deficiency in pregnancy
- Contains 33% elemental iron
- Keep upright for 15–30 minutes to avoid esophageal corrosion; take 1 hour before bedtime
- Stools will become black or dark green
- Notify clinician if stools are tarry or blood-streaked; indicates GI bleeding
- Do not substitute one iron salt for another because iron content differs
- Give 1 hour before or 2 hours after meals
- Liquid may stain teeth
- Do not take within 1 hour before or 2 hours after antacids, eggs, whole-grain bread or cereal, milk, coffee, or tea
- Rx

• •

SIDE EFFECTS

Nausea, constipation   Black or discolored stools
Epigastric pain

NURSING CONSIDERATIONS

- Treatment of iron deficiency anemia, prophylaxis for iron deficiency in pregnancy
- Contains 12% elemental iron
- Keep upright for 15–30 minutes to avoid esophageal corrosion; take 1 hour before bedtime
- Stools will become black or dark green
- Notify clinician if stools are tarry or blood-streaked; indicates GI bleeding
- Take on empty stomach, if possible
- Do not substitute one iron salt for another because iron content differs
- Liquid may stain teeth
- Do not take 1 hour before or 2 hours after antacids, eggs, whole-grain bread or cereal, milk, coffee, or tea
- Rx

FERROUS SULFATE
(Feosol)

• •

IRON POLYSACCHARIDE
(Niferex)

SIDE EFFECTS

Nausea, constipation   Black or discolored stools
Epigastric pain

NURSING CONSIDERATIONS

- Treatment of iron deficiency anemia, prophylaxis for iron deficiency in pregnancy
- Contains 30% elemental iron
- Keep upright for 15–30 minutes to avoid esophageal corrosion; take 1 hour before bedtime
- Stools will become black or dark green
- Notify clinician if stools are tarry or blood-streaked; indicates GI bleeding
- May be taken with or without food
- Do not substitute one iron salt for another because iron content differs
- Liquid may stain teeth
- Do not take within 1 hour or 2 hours after antacids, eggs, whole-grain bread or cereal, milk, coffee, or tea
- Rx

• •

SIDE EFFECTS

Nausea, constipation   Black or discolored stools
Epigastric pain

NURSING CONSIDERATIONS

- Treatment of iron deficiency anemia, prophylaxis for iron deficiency in pregnancy
- Keep upright for 15–30 minutes to avoid esophageal corrosion; take 1 hour before bedtime
- Stools will become black or dark green
- Notify clinician if stools are tarry or blood-streaked; indicates GI bleeding
- Take on empty stomach, if possible; may be taken with food
- Do not substitute one iron salt for another because iron content differs
- Liquid may stain teeth
- Do not take within 1 hour or 2 hours after antacids, eggs, whole-grain bread or cereal, milk, coffee, or tea
- Rx

POTASSIUM

. . . .

NALOXONE HCL
(nal-<u>ox</u>-own)

SIDE EFFECTS

Nausea, vomiting   Cramps, diarrhea

NURSING CONSIDERATIONS

- Prevention and treatment of hypokalemia
- PO: onset 30 minutes; give while patient is sitting up or standing
- IV: onset immediate
- Do not infuse faster than 10 mg/hr in adults
- Do not give IM, subQ, IV push
- Dilute liquid prior to giving via NG
- Monitor IV infusions for extravasation: IV infusions may sting or burn
- Report hyperkalemia: lethargy, confusion, GI symptoms, fainting, decreased urinary output
- Report continued hypokalemia: fatigue, weakness, polyuria, polydipsia, cardiac changes
- Avoid OTC antacids, salt substitutes, analgesics, vitamins unless directed by clinician
- OTC, Rx

● ●

SIDE EFFECTS

Withdrawal symptoms in narcotic-dependent patients: restlessness, muscle spasms, tearing

NURSING CONSIDERATIONS

- Used to reverse narcotic depression, including respiratory symptoms
- IM and subQ onset in 2–5 minutes; IV 1–2 minutes
- Have emergency support equipment available
- May increase PTT
- Monitor for bleeding in surgical and obstetric patients
- Rx

ERGOCALCIFEROL
(er-goe-kal-<u>sif</u>-e-role)

(Vitamin D2)

• •

CYANOCOBALAMIN
(sye-an-oh-koe-<u>bal</u>-a-min)

(Vitamin B12)

SIDE EFFECTS

Metallic taste, dry mouth
Hypervitaminosis D

NURSING CONSIDERATIONS

- Treatment of vitamin D deficiency, rickets, psoriasis, rheumatoid arthritis, hypoparathyroidism
- If med is missed, omit
- Decrease use of antacids and laxatives containing magnesium
- Mineral oil interferes with absorption
- Rx

● ●

SIDE EFFECTS

Diarrhea

NURSING CONSIDERATIONS

- Treatment of vitamin B12 deficiency, pernicious anemia, hemorrhage, renal and hepatic disease
- IM, subQ, nasal: peak 3–10 days
- Foods high in this vitamin: meats, seafood, egg yolk, fermented cheeses
- Excessive intake of alcohol or vitamin C may decrease oral absorption/effectiveness
- OTC, Rx

FOLIC ACID
(<u>foe</u>-lik <u>a</u>-cid)

HYDROXOCOBALAMIN
(hye-<u>drox</u>-o-ko-bal-a-min)

(Vitamin B12)

SIDE EFFECTS

Bronchospasm
Hypersensitivity

NURSING CONSIDERATIONS

- Treatment of anemia, liver disease, alcoholism, intestinal obstruction, folic acid deficiency, esp. in pregnant women
- Also contained in bran, yeast, dried beans, nuts, fruits, fresh vegetables, asparagus
- OTC

. . . .

SIDE EFFECTS

Diarrhea
Hypersensitivity

NURSING CONSIDERATIONS

- Treatment of vitamin B12 deficiency, pernicious anemia, hemorrhage, renal and hepatic disease
- IM, subQ: peak 3–10 days
- Foods high in this vitamin: meats, seafood, egg yolk, fermented cheeses
- OTC, Rx

DTAP VACCINE
(<u>dee</u>-tap vak-<u>seen</u>)

(Infanrix, Tripedia, Daptacel)

• •

HAEMOPHILUS INFLUENZAE TYPE B (HIB) VACCINE
(he-<u>mah</u>-fill-us tipe bee vak-<u>seen</u>)

(ActHib, PedVaxHib, Hiberix)

Side Effects

Fever (25%)

Redness or swelling at injection site (25%)

Soreness at injection site (25%)

Fussiness (33%)

Serious allergic reaction in less than 1 per 1 million doses

Nursing Considerations

- Used to prevent diphtheria, tetanus (lockjaw), and acellular pertussis (whooping cough)
- Contains only portions of the bacteria; cannot cause infection
- Control fever with aspirin-free pain reliever, esp. in child with seizures
- Children: administer in 5 doses

• •

Side Effects

Injection site redness, warmth (uncommon)

Dizziness, shoulder pain (very rare)

Nursing Considerations

- Used to prevent bacterial meningitis and other infections in children under age 5
- Contains only portions of the bacteria; cannot cause infection
- Children: administer in 3 or 4 doses (depends on brand)

HEPATITIS A VACCINE

(hep-uh-<u>tye</u>-tis aay vak-<u>seen</u>)

(Vaqta, Havrix)

. . . .

HEPATITIS B VACCINE

(hep-uh-<u>tye</u>-tis bee vak-<u>seen</u>)

(Recombivax HB, Engerix)

Side Effects

Soreness at injection site
(50% in adults, 17% in
children)

Headache (17% in adults, 4% in
children)
Serious allergic reaction rare

Nursing Considerations

- Used to prevent serious liver disease
- Contains the whole, but killed virus; cannot cause infection
- 2 doses needed for lasting protection

· ·

Side Effects

Soreness at injection site (25%)
Severe allergic reaction in 1 per 1.1 million doses

Nursing Considerations

- Used to prevent liver infection
- Contains only portions of virus; cannot cause infection
- Infants: administer in 3 doses

HUMAN PAPILLOMAVIRUS (HPV) VACCINE

(<u>hyoo</u>-man pap-ill-<u>oh</u>-mah-<u>vye</u>-rus vak-<u>seen</u>)

(Cervarix for women, Gardasil for both men and women)

• •

INFLUENZA VACCINE

(in-floo-<u>en</u>-zuh vak-<u>seen</u>)

(Fluzone, Flumist nasal spray)

Side Effects

Pain at injection site (90% for Cervarix, 80% for Gardisil)

Redness or swelling (50% for Cervarix, 25% for Gardisil)

Headache or fatigue (50% for Cervarix, 33% for Gardisil)

GI symptoms (25% for Cervarix)

Muscle or joint pain (50% for Cervarix)

Nursing Considerations

- Used to prevent sexually transmitted diseases that cause cervical cancer in women
- Contains only portions of the virus; cannot cause infection
- Cervarix recommended for girls age 11–12; Gardasil recommended for girls and boys age 11–12
- Given as 3-dose series

• •

Side Effects

Injection-site swelling, soreness

Flulike symptoms (nasal spray)

Nursing Considerations

- Used to prevent influenza infection
- IM: injection contains the whole but killed virus; cannot cause infection
- Nasal spray: contains live, weakened viruses; designed to trigger a mild infection, inducing immunity
- Serious allergic reaction in less than 1 per 1 million doses

MEASLES, MUMPS, & RUBELLA (MMR) VACCINE
(<u>mee</u>-zulls mumps and roo-<u>bell</u>-uh vak-<u>seen</u>)

(M-M-R II)

• •

MENINGOCOCCAL VACCINE
(men-in-go-<u>cok</u>-ull vak-<u>seen</u>)

(Menactra, Menveo)

Side Effects
Fever (17%)

Nursing Considerations
- Used to prevent infection with measles, mumps, and rubella ("German measles")
- Contains live but weakened viruses; can cause the actual diseases
- Serious allergic reactions in less than 1 in 1 million doses
- Children: administer in 2 doses

• •

Side Effects
Redness or pain at injection site (50%)

Nursing Considerations
- Used to prevent 4 types of bacterial meningitis, including 2 of the 3 types most common in United States
- Contains only portions of the bacteria; cannot cause infection
- Adolescents: 2 doses recommended
- Serious allergic reactions very rare

PNEUMOCOCCAL CONJUGATE (PCV13) VACCINE
(<u>new</u>-moe-cok-ull <u>con</u>-juh-get vak-<u>seen</u>)

(Prevnar)

• •

POLIO VACCINE
(<u>poe</u>-lee-oh vak-<u>seen</u>)

(IPOL)

Side Effects

Children: drowsiness, anorexia, injection-site redness or tenderness (50%)
Children: irritability (80%)

Children: mild fever, swelling at injection site (33%)
Adults: mild reactions

Nursing Considerations

- Used to prevent infection by Streptococcus pneumoniae bacteria
- PCV13 vaccine protects against 13 of the more than 90 types of pneumococcal bacteria
- PPSV23 vaccine (given to adults over age 65) protects against 23 strains of pneumococcal bacteria
- Contains only portions of the bacteria; cannot cause disease

● ●

Side Effects

Mild fever
Injection-site soreness

Extremely small risk of allergic reaction

Nursing Considerations

- Used to prevent paralysis and meningitis
- Contains whole but killed virus; cannot cause disease
- Children: administer in 4 doses

ROTAVIRUS VACCINE
(<u>row</u>-ta-vye-rus vak-<u>seen</u>)

(Rotateq, Rotarix)

· ·

VARICELLA VACCINE
(<u>vair</u>-i-sell-ah vak-<u>seen</u>)

(Varivax for childhood disease, Zostavax for shingles)

Side Effects

Irritability
GI upset

Nursing Considerations

- Prevents infection with a virus that causes diarrhea and other GI problems
- Contains the whole live virus; designed to trigger low-grade infection to create immunity
- Administer PO: oral liquid vaccine
- Infants: administer in 2 or 3 doses (depends on brand)

• •

Side Effects

Soreness at injection site   Rash (rare)
Fever

Nursing Considerations

- Varivax used to prevent infection with the varicella (chickenpox) virus, which causes diarrhea and other GI problems in babies and young children; Zostavax used to prevent shingles (zoster) in adults age 60 or older
- Both injections contain live, but weakened virus; immunization can cause a mild case of the disease
- Counsel patient to avoid contact with newborns, pregnant women, and immunocompromised individuals immediately after injection

DESOGESTREL/ ETHINYL ESTRADIOL
(dess-oh-<u>jes</u>-trel/<u>eth</u>-in-il es-tra-<u>dye</u>-ole)

(Desogen, Mircette, Ortho-Cept)

• •

DROSPIRENONE/ ETHINYL ESTRADIOL
(dro-<u>spy</u>-re-noan/<u>eth</u>-in-il es-tra-<u>dye</u>-ole)

(Yaz)

SIDE EFFECTS

Headache   Dizziness
Breakthrough bleeding, spotting Nausea
Contact lens intolerance

NURSING CONSIDERATIONS

- Prevention of pregnancy, treatment of endometriosis, hypermenorrhea (monophasic)
- Counsel patient to contact clinician if unusual bleeding, severe headache, difficulty breathing, changes in vision/coordination, chest/leg pain
- Counsel patient this medication does not protect against STDs or HIV
- Avoid smoking, which increases risk of adverse cardiovascular events
- Stop med for at least 1 week before surgery to decrease risk of thromboembolism
- St. John's wort may decrease effectiveness
- Rx

• •

SIDE EFFECTS

Headache   Painful menstrual   Weakness
Breast pain   period, menstrual   URI
Vaginal itching,   disorder, break-   Weight gain
   discharge, or yeast   through bleeding   Symptoms of
   infection   Increase in BP   depression
Nausea   Sinusitis   UTI

NURSING CONSIDERATIONS

- Used to prevent pregnancy, treatment for PMDD and moderate acne vulgaris
- Take at the same time daily, once a day
- Avoid smoking, which increases risk of adverse cardiovascular events
- Counsel patient this medication does not protect against STDs or HIV
- Teach patient to promptly report any visual disturbances, unusual bleeding, chest or leg pain, change in coordination, dyspnea, or severe headache
- Monitor BP
- May increase risk of cardiovascular events including MI and stroke
- St. John's wort may decrease effectiveness
- Rx

ETHINYL ESTRADIOL/ ETHYNODIOL
(eth-in-il es-tra-<u>dye</u>-ole/e-thi-noe-<u>dye</u>-ole

(Demulen)

● ●

ETHINYL ESTRADIOL/ NORETHINDRONE
(eth-in-il es-tra-<u>dye</u>-ole/nor-eth-<u>in</u>-drone)

(Ortho-Novum 7-7-7)

SIDE EFFECTS

Headache
Breakthrough bleeding, spotting
Dizziness

Nausea
Contact lens intolerance

NURSING CONSIDERATIONS

- Prevention of pregnancy (monophasic contraceptive), treatment of endometriosis, hypermenorrhea
- Counsel patient this medication does not protect against STDs or HIV
- Contact clinician if unusual bleeding, severe headache, difficulty breathing, changes in vision/coordination, chest/leg pain
- Avoid smoking, which increases risk of adverse cardiovascular events
- Stop med for at least 1 week before surgery to decrease risk of thromboembolism
- St. John's wort may decrease effectiveness
- Rx

. . . .

SIDE EFFECTS

Nausea
Bloating
Headache

Breakthrough bleeding
Contact lens intolerance
Dizziness

NURSING CONSIDERATIONS

- Female contraception (triphasic);
- Counsel patient this medication does not protect against STDs or HIV
- Contact clinician if breast lumps, vaginal bleeding, edema, jaundice, dark urine, clay-colored stools, dyspnea, headache, blurred vision, abdominal pain, numbness or stiffness in legs, chest pain, tenderness with redness and swelling in extremities
- Contact clinician if weekly weight gain is over 5 pounds
- Can take with food or milk to decrease GI upset
- St. John's wort may decrease effectiveness
- Rx

MESTRANOL/
NORETHINDRONE
(<u>mes</u>-tre-nole/nor-eth-<u>in</u>-drone)

(Norinyl)

• •

NORETHINDRONE
(nor-eth-<u>in</u>-drone)

(Micronor, Nor-Qd)

SIDE EFFECTS

Headache

Breakthrough bleeding, spotting

Contact lens intolerance

Dizziness

Nausea

NURSING CONSIDERATIONS

- Prevention of pregnancy (monophasic contraception), treatment of endometriosis, hypermenorrhea
- Counsel patient this medication does not protect against STDs or HIV
- Contact clinician if unusual bleeding, severe headache, difficult breathing, changes in vision/coordination, chest/leg pain
- Avoid smoking, which increases risk of adverse cardiovascular events
- Stop med for at least 1 week before surgery to decrease risk of thromboembolism
- St. John's wort may decrease effectiveness
- Rx

• •

SIDE EFFECTS

Nausea

Headache

Irregular bleeding (genital)

NURSING CONSIDERATIONS

- Management of abnormal uterine bleeding, amenorrhea, endometriosis, contraception
- Counsel patient this medication does not protect against STDs or HIV
- Contact clinician if breast lumps, vaginal bleeding, edema, jaundice, dark urine, clay-colored stools, dyspnea, headache, blurred vision, abdominal pain, numbness or stiffness in legs, chest pain, tenderness with redness and swelling in extremities
- Contact clinician if weekly weight gain is over 5 pounds
- Can take with food or milk to decrease GI upset
- Cigarette smoking increases risk of serious cardiovascular disease
- Rx

ESTRADIOL (ORAL)
(es-tra-<u>dye</u>-ole)

(Estrace)

· ·

ESTRADIOL CYPIONATE, ESTRADIOL VALERATE
(es-tra-<u>dye</u>-ole)

(Depogen, Delestrogen, Valergen)

SIDE EFFECTS

Nausea   Testicular atrophy
Gynecomastia   Impotence
Contact lens intolerance   Headache

NURSING CONSIDERATIONS

- Treatment of symptoms of menopause, inoperable breast cancer (selected cases), prostatic cancer, atrophic vaginitis, prevention of osteoporosis
- Contact clinician if breast lumps, vaginal bleeding, edema, jaundice, dark urine, clay-colored stools, dyspnea, headache, blurred vision, abdominal pain, numbness or stiffness in legs, chest pain, tenderness with redness and swelling in extremities
- Men should contact clinician to report impotence or gynecomastia
- Contact clinician if weekly weight gain is over 5 pounds
- Can take with food or milk to decrease GI upset
- May increase risk of endometrial cancer
- May increase risk of cardiovascular events
- Rx

• •

SIDE EFFECTS

Contact lens intolerance   Testicular atrophy
Gynecomastia   Impotence

NURSING CONSIDERATIONS

- Treatment of symptoms of menopause, inoperable breast cancer (selected cases), prostatic cancer, atrophic vaginitis, prevention of osteoporosis
- IM: inject deep into large muscle mass
- Contact clinician if breast lumps, vaginal bleeding, edema, jaundice, dark urine, clay-colored stools, dyspnea, headache, blurred vision, abdominal pain, numbness or stiffness in legs, chest pain, tenderness with redness and swelling in extremities
- Men should contact clinician to report impotence or gynecomastia
- Contact clinician if weekly weight gain is over 5 pounds
- May increase risk of cardiovascular events
- Rx

ESTRADIOL PATCH
(es-tra-<u>dye</u>-ole)

(Alora, Climara, Estraderm, FemPatch)

• •

ESTROGENS CONJUGATED
(<u>ess</u>-troh-genz)

(Premarin)

SIDE EFFECTS

Contact lens intolerance   Testicular atrophy
Gynecomastia   Impotence

NURSING CONSIDERATIONS

- Treatment of symptoms of menopause, inoperable breast cancer (selected cases), prostatic cancer, atrophic vaginitis, prevention of osteoporosis
- Apply patch to trunk of body twice a week; press firmly and hold in place for 10 seconds to ensure good contact
- Contact clinician if breast lumps, vaginal bleeding, edema, jaundice, dark urine, clay-colored stools, dyspnea, headache, blurred vision, abdominal pain, numbness or stiffness in legs, chest pain, tenderness with redness and swelling in extremities
- Men should contact clinician to report impotence or gynecomastia
- Contact clinician if weekly weight gain is over 5 pounds
- May increase risk of cardiovascular events
- May increase risk of endometrial cancer
- May impair GTT results
- Rx

. . . .

SIDE EFFECTS

Nausea   Testicular atrophy
Gynecomastia   Impotence
Contact lens intolerance

NURSING CONSIDERATIONS

- Treatment of symptoms of menopause, inoperable breast cancer, prostatic cancer, abnormal uterine bleeding, prevention of osteoporosis
- IM: inject deep into large muscle mass
- PO: can take with food or milk to decrease GI upset
- Contact clinician if breast lumps, vaginal bleeding, edema, jaundice, dark urine, clay-colored stools, dyspnea, headache, blurred vision, abdominal pain, numbness or stiffness in legs, chest pain, tenderness with redness and swelling in extremities
- Men should contact clinician to report impotence or gynecomastia
- Contact clinician if weekly weight gain is over 5 pounds
- May increase risk of cardiovascular events
- May increase risk of endometrial cancer
- May increase risk of ovarian cancer
- Rx

CLOMIPHENE CITRATE
(<u>klo</u>-mi-feen <u>sye</u>-trate)

(Clomid, Serophene)

. . . .

Women's Health
Progestins

MEDROXYPROGESTERONE ACETATE
(me-drox-ee-proe-<u>jess</u>-te-rone)

(Provera, Depo-Provera)

SIDE EFFECTS

Vasomotor flushes
Breast discomfort
Heavy menses
Mental depression
Headache
Nausea, vomiting
Increased appetite, weight gain

Constipation, bloating
Spontaneous abortion
Multiple ovulations
Enlarged ovaries with multiple
   follicular cysts
Ophthalmic "floaters," diplopia

NURSING CONSIDERATIONS

- Fertility drug to stimulate ovulation
- Teach patient to report abnormal bleeding immediately
- Monitor for visual disturbances
- Teach patient to report pelvic pain immediately
- Teach patient to report menopause-like symptoms immediately
- Teach patient to report weight gain or edema or decreased urination immediately
- Patient should stop medication if pregnancy is suspected
- Rx

· ·

SIDE EFFECTS

Nausea
Contact lens intolerance
Testicular atrophy

Impotence
GI upset
Galactorrhea

NURSING CONSIDERATIONS

- Management of abnormal uterine bleeding, secondary amenorrhea, endometrial cancer, renal cancer, contraceptive, prevent endometrial changes associated with estrogen replacement therapy
- IM: inject deep into large muscle mass, rotate sites, injection may be painful
- Counsel patient this medication does not protect against STDs or HIV
- Contact clinician if weekly weight gain is over 5 pounds
- Use with caution with history of depression
- Contact clinician if swelling in calves, sudden chest pain, or SOB
- May increase risk of cardiovascular events
- May increase risk of ovarian and breast cancer
- May impair glucose metabolism; monitor blood sugars in diabetic patients
- Rx

APPENDIX A:

Controlled Substance Schedules

Drugs regulated by the Controlled Substances Act of 1970 are classified:

Schedule I: High abuse potential and no accepted medical use. Examples include heroin, marijuana, peyote, Ecstasy, and LSD.

Schedule II: High abuse potential with severe dependence liability. Examples include narcotics, amphetamines, and some barbiturates.

Schedule III: Less abuse potential than schedule II drugs and moderate dependence liability. Examples include nonbarbiturate sedatives, nonamphetamine stimulants, anabolic steroids, and limited amounts of certain narcotics.

Schedule IV: Less abuse potential than schedule III drugs and limited dependence liability. Examples include some sedatives, anxiolytics, and nonnarcotic analgesics.

Schedule V: Limited abuse potential. Examples include small amounts of narcotics, such as codeine, used as antidiarrheals or antitussives.

APPENDIX B:

Special Considerations

Black box warning, also known as boxed warning: Food and Drug Administration (FDA) warning placed by the manufacturer on a prescription drug package insert. It communicates that the medication carries a significant risk of serious or even life-threatening adverse effects.

Off-label use: Use of medications for an unapproved indication or in an unapproved age group, unapproved dosage, or unapproved route of administration.

Pregnancy and lactation: Prior to June 2015, the FDA required that most prescribed medications be labeled for risk according to letter categories A (remote possibility of fetal harm), B, C, D, and X (studies show evidence of fetal risk). Beginning in June 2015, the FDA changed to a system in which health care providers assess the benefit versus the risk of a given medication for individual pregnant women and nursing mothers. FDA guidelines call for subsequent counseling of pregnant and lactating patients, "allowing them to make informed and educated decisions for themselves and their children." The FDA created a pregnancy exposure registry to collect and maintain data on the effects of approved drugs that are prescribed to and used by pregnant women (FDA *Pregnancy and Lactation Labeling Final Rule*, December 3, 2014).

APPENDIX C:

Common Medical Abbreviations

ABC—airway, breathing, circulation

abd.—abdomen

ABG—arterial blood gas

ABO—system of classifying blood groups

ac—before meals

ACE—angiotensin-converting enzyme

ACS—acute compartment syndrome

ACTH—adrenocorticotrophic hormone

ADH—antidiuretic hormone

ADHD—attention deficit hyperactivity disorder

ADL—activities of daily living

ad lib—freely, as desired

AFP—alpha-fetoprotein

AIDS—acquired immunodeficiency syndrome

AKA—above-the-knee amputation

ALL—acute lymphocytic leukemia

ALS—amyotrophic lateral sclerosis

ALT—alkaline phosphatase (formerly SGPT)

AMI—antibody-mediated immunity

AML—acute myelogenous leukemia

amt.—amount

ANA—antinuclear antibody

ANS—autonomic nervous system

AP—anteroposterior

A&P—anterior and posterior

APC—atrial premature contraction

aq.—water

ARDS—adult respiratory distress syndrome

ASD—atrial septal defect

ASHD—atherosclerotic heart disease

AST—aspartate aminotransferase (formerly SGOT)

ATP—adenosine triphosphate

AV—atrioventricular

BCG—Bacille Calmette-Guerin

bid—two times a day

BKA—below-the-knee amputation

BLS—basic life support

BMR—basal metabolic rate

BP—blood pressure

BPH—benign prostatic hypertrophy

bpm—beats per minute

BPR—bathroom privileges

BSA—body surface area

BUN—blood, urea, nitrogen

C—centigrade, Celsius

c—with

Ca—calcium

CA—cancer

CABG—coronary artery bypass graft

CAD—coronary artery disease

CAPD—continuous ambulatory peritoneal dialysis

caps—capsules

CBC—complete blood count

CC—chief complaint

CCU—coronary care unit, critical care unit

CDC—Centers for Disease Control and Prevention

CHF—congestive heart failure

CK—creatine kinase

Cl—chloride

CLL—chronic lymphocytic leukemia

cm—centimeter

CMV—cytomegalovirus infection

CNS—central nervous system

CO—carbon monoxide, cardiac output

CO2—carbon dioxide

comp—compound

cont—continuous

COPD—chronic obstructive pulmonary disease

CP—cerebral palsy

CPAP—continuous positive airway pressure

CPK—creatine phosphokinase

CPR—cardiopulmonary resuscitation

CRP—C-reactive protein

C&S—culture and sensitivity

CSF—cerebrospinal fluid

CT—computed tomography

CTD—connective tissue disease

CTS—carpal tunnel syndrome

cu—cubic

CVA—cerebrovascular accident or costovertebral angle

CVC—central venous catheter

CVP—central venous pressure

D&C—dilation and curettage

DIC—disseminated intravascular coagulation

DIFF—differential blood count

dil.—dilute

DJD—degenerative joint disease

DKA—diabetic ketoacidosis

dL—deciliter (100 mL)

DM—diabetes mellitus

DNA—deoxyribonucleic acid

DNR—do not resuscitate

DO—doctor of osteopathy

DOE—dyspnea on exertion

DPT—vaccine for diphtheria, pertussis, tetanus

Dr.—doctor

DVT—deep vein thrombosis

D/W—dextrose in water

Dx—diagnosis

ECF—extracellular fluid

ECG or EKG—electrocardiogram

ECT—electroconvulsive therapy

ED—emergency department

EEG—electroencephalogram

EMD—electromechanical dissociation

EMG—electromyography

ENT—ear, nose, and throat

ESR—erythrocyte sedimentation rate

ESRD—end stage renal disease

ET—endotracheal tube

F—Fahrenheit

FBD—fibrocystic breast disease

FBS—fasting blood sugar

FDA—U.S. Food and Drug Administration

FFP—fresh frozen plasma

fl—fluid

4 x 4—piece of gauze 4 inches long by 4 inches wide used for dressings

FSH—follicle-stimulating hormone

ft.—foot, feet (unit of measure)

FUO—fever of undetermined origin

g—gram

GB—gallbladder

GFR—glomerular filtration rate

GH—growth hormone

GI—gastrointestinal

gr—grain

GSC—Glasgow coma scale

GTT—glucose tolerance test

gtts—drops

GU—genitourinary

GYN—gynecological

h or hrs—hour or hours

(H)—hypodermically

Hb or Hgb—hemoglobin

hCG—human chorionic gonadotropin

HCO3-—bicarbonate

Hct—hematocrit

HD—hemodialysis

HDL—high-density lipoproteins

Hg—mercury

Hgb—hemoglobin

HGH—human growth hormone

HHNC—hyperglycemia hyperosmolar nonketotic coma

HIV—human immunodeficiency virus

HLA—human leukocyte antigen

HR—heart rate
hr—hour
HSV—herpes simplex virus
HTN—hypertension
H₂O—water
Hx—history
Hz—hertz (cycles/second)
IAPB—intraaortic balloon pump
IBS—irritable bowel syndrome
ICF—intracellular fluid
ICP—intracranial pressure
ICS—intercostal space
ICU—intensive care unit
IDDM—insulin-dependent diabetes mellitus
IgA—immunoglobulin A
IM—intramuscular
I&O—intake and output
IOP—intraocular pressure
IPG—impedance plethysmogram
IPPB—intermittent positive-pressure breathing
IUD—intrauterine device
IV—intravenous
IVC—intraventricular catheter
IVP—intravenous pyelogram
JRA—juvenile rheumatoid arthritis
K⁺—potassium
kcal—kilocalorie (food calorie)

kg—kilogram
KO, KVO—keep vein open
KS—Kaposi sarcoma
KUB—kidneys, ureters, bladder
L, l—liter
lab—laboratory
lb—pound
LBBB—left bundle branch block
LDH—lactate dehydrogenase
LDL—low-density lipoproteins
LE—lupus erythematosus
LH—luteinizing hormone
liq—liquid
LLQ—left lower quadrant
LOC—level of consciousness
LP—lumbar puncture
LPN, LVN—licensed practical or vocational nurse
LTC—long-term care
LUQ—left upper quadrant
LV—left ventricle
m—minim, meter, micron
MAOI—monoamine oxidase inhibitor
MAST—military antishock trousers
mcg—microgram
MCH—mean corpuscular hemoglobin
MCV—mean corpuscular volume

MD—muscular dystrophy, medical doctor

MDI—metered dose inhaler

mEq—milliequivalent

mg—milligram

Mg—magnesium

MG—myasthenia gravis

MI—myocardial infarction

mL—milliliter

mm—millimeter

MMR—vaccine for measles, mumps, and rubella

MRI—magnetic resonance imaging

MS—multiple sclerosis

N—nitrogen, normal (strength of solution)

NIDDM—non-insulin-dependent diabetes mellitus

Na+—sodium

NaCl—sodium chloride

NANDA—North American Nursing Diagnosis Association

NG—nasogastric

NGT—nasogastric tube

NLN—National League for Nursing

noc—at night

NPO—nothing by mouth

NS—normal saline

NSR—normal sinus rhythm (cardiac)

NSAIDs—nonsteroidal antiinflammatory drugs

NSNA—National Student Nurses' Association

NST—nonstress test

O₂—oxygen

OB-GYN—obstetrics and gynecology

OCT—oxytocin challenge test

OOB—out of bed

OPC—outpatient clinic

OR—operating room

os—by mouth

OSHA—Occupational Safety and Health Administration

OTC—over-the-counter (drug that can be obtained without a prescription)

oz—ounce

p—with

P—pulse, pressure, phosphorus

PA chest—posterior-anterior chest x-ray

PAC—premature atrial complexes

PaCO₂—partial pressure of carbon dioxide in arterial blood

PaO₂—partial pressure of oxygen in arterial blood

PAD—peripheral artery disease

Pap—Papanicolaou smear

PBI—protein-bound iodine

pc—after meals

PCA—patient-controlled analgesia

PCO$_2$—partial pressure of carbon dioxide

PCP—*Pneumocystis jiroveci* pneumonia (formerly *Pneumocystis carinii* pneumonia)

PD—peritoneal dialysis

PE—pulmonary embolism

PEEP—positive end-expiratory pressure

PERRLA—pupils equal, round, reactive to light and accommodation

PET—postural emission tomography

PFT—pulmonary function tests

pH—hydrogen ion concentration

PID—pelvic inflammatory disease

PKD—polycystic disease

PKU—phenylketonuria

PMDD—premenstrual dysphoric disorder

PMS—premenstrual syndrome

PND—paroxysmal nocturnal dyspnea

PO, po—by mouth

PO$_2$—partial pressure of oxygen

PPD—positive purified protein derivative (of tuberculin)

PPN—partial parenteral nutrition

PRN, prn—as needed, whenever necessary

pro time—prothrombin time

PSA—prostate-specific antigen

psi—pounds per square inch

PSP—phenolsulfonphthalein

PT—physical therapy, prothrombin time

PTCA—percutaneous transluminal coronary angioplasty

PTH—parathyroid hormone

PTT—partial thromboplastin time

PUD—peptic ulcer disease

PVC—premature ventricular contraction

q—every

QA—quality assurance

qh—every hour

q 2 h—every 2 hours

q 4 h—every 4 hours

qid—four times a day

qs—quantity sufficient

R—rectal temperature, respirations, roentgen

RA—rheumatoid arthritis

RAI—radioactive iodine

RAIU—radioactive iodine uptake

RAS—reticular activating system

RBBB—right bundle branch block

RBC—red blood cell or count

RCA—right coronary artery

RDA—recommended dietary allowance

resp—respirations

RF—rheumatic fever, rheumatoid factor

Rh—antigen on blood cell indicated by + or –

RIND—reversible ischemic neurologic deficit

RLQ—right lower quadrant

RN—registered nurse

RNA—ribonucleic acid

R/O, r/o—rule out, to exclude

ROM—range of motion (of joint)

RUQ—right upper quadrant

Rx—prescription

s—without

S. or Sig.—(Signa) to write on label

SA—sinoatrial node

SaO$_2$—systemic arterial oxygen saturation (%)

sat sol—saturated solution

SBE—subacute bacterial endocarditis

SDA—same-day admission

SDS—same-day surgery

sed rate—sedimentation rate

SGOT—serum glutamic-oxaloacetic transaminase (see AST)

SGPT—serum glutamic-pyruvic transaminase (see ALT)

SI—International System of Units

SIADH—syndrome of inappropriate antidiuretic hormone

SIDS—sudden infant death syndrome

SL—sublingual

SLE—systemic lupus erythematosus

SOB—short of breath

sol—solution

SMBG—self-monitoring blood glucose

SMR—submucous resection

sp gr—specific gravity

spec.—specimen

SSKI—saturated solution of potassium iodide

stat—immediately

STI—sexually transmitted infection

subcut, SubQ—subcutaneous

Sx—symptoms

Syr.—syrup

T—temperature, thoracic (to be followed by the number designating specific thoracic vertebra)

T&A—tonsillectomy and adenoidectomy

tabs—tablets

TB—tuberculosis

T&C—type and crossmatch

TED—thromboembolic device (compression stockings)

temp—temperature

TENS—transcutaneous electrical nerve stimulation

TIA—transient ischemic attack

TIBC—total iron binding capacity

tid—three times a day

tinct, or tr.—tincture

TMJ—temporomandibular joint

tPA, TPA—tissue plasminogen activator

TPN—total parenteral nutrition

TPR—temperature, pulse, respiration

TQM—total quality management

TSE—testicular self-examination

TSH—thyroid-stimulating hormone

tsp—teaspoon

TSS—toxic shock syndrome

TURP—transurethral prostatectomy

UA—urinalysis

ung—ointment

URI—upper respiratory tract infection

UTI—urinary tract infection

VAD—venous access device

VDRL—Venereal Disease Research Laboratory (test for syphilis)

VF, Vfib—ventricular fibrillation

VPC—ventricular premature complexes

VS, vs—vital signs

VSD—ventricular septal defect

VT—ventricular tachycardia

WBC—white blood cell or count

WHO—World Health Organization

wt—weight

BRAND NAME DRUG INDEX

Librium (chlordiazepoxide), 187

Lidex (fluocinonide), 131

Lioresal (baclofen), 227

Lipitor (atorvastatin calcium), 95

Lithobid (lithium), 213

Lopressor (metoprolol tartrate), 107

Lortab (hydrocodone bitartrate/acetaminophen), 17

Lotensin (benazepril hydrochloride), 73

Lovenox (enoxaparin), 25

Luminal (phenobarbital), 33

Lyrica (pregabalin), 35

Macrobid (nitrofurantoin), 179

Macrodantin (nitrofurantoin), 179

Maxipime (cefepime), 53

Maxzide (hydrochlorothiazide/ triamterene), 121

Medrol (methylprednisolone), 65

Menactra (meningococcal vaccine), 283

Menveo (meningococcal vaccine), 283

Methadose (methadone), 21

Meticorten (prednisone), 67

Mevacor (lovastatin), 99

Micronor (norethindrone), 293

Microzide (hydrochlorothiazide), 125

Minipress (prazosin hydrochloride), 79

Minocin (minocycline hydrochloride), 63

Mircette (desogestrel/ethinyl estradiol), 289

M-M-R II (measles, mumps, and rubella vaccine), 283

Motrin IB (ibuprofen), 15, 69, 221

MS Contin (morphine), 21

Mucinex (guaifenesin), 261

Mycostatin (nystatin), 129

Myproic Acid (valproic acid), 37

Mytussin (guaifenesin), 261

Namenda XR (memantine hydrochloride), 237

Naprosyn (naproxen sodium), 15, 71, 223

Nasacort AQ Spray (triamcinolone), 9

NasalCrom (cromolyn sodium), 261

Nasalide (flunisolide), 5

Nasonex Spray (mometasone), 9

Neurontin (gabapentin), 31

Nexium (esomeprazole magnesium), 157

Niacor (niacin), 99

Niaspan (niacin), 99

Niferex (iron polysaccharide), 269

Nitro-Par (nitroglycerin), 85

GENERIC NAME DRUG INDEX